# Health Care Reform
# and Disparities

# Health Care Reform and Disparities

## History, Hype, and Hope

Toni P. Miles

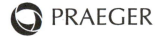

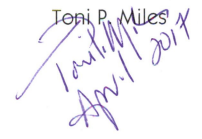

PRAEGER

AN IMPRINT OF ABC-CLIO, LLC
Santa Barbara, California • Denver, Colorado • Oxford, England

**Library of Congress Cataloging-in-Publication Data**

Miles, Toni P.
  Health care reform and disparities : history, hype, and hope / Toni P. Miles.
      p. ; cm.
  Includes bibliographical references and index.
  ISBN 978-0-313-39768-4 (hardback : alk. paper) — ISBN 978-0-313-39769-1
(e-book)
  I.  Title.
  [DNLM: 1.   Healthcare Disparities—United States. 2.   Health Care Reform—
United States. 3.   Insurance, Health—United States.   W 84 AA1]
  LC   Classification not assigned
  368.38'2—dc23        2012008765

ISBN: 978-0-313-39768-4
EISBN: 978-0-313-39769-1

16   15   14                          4   5

This book is also available on the World Wide Web as an eBook.
Visit www.abc-clio.com for details.

Praeger
An Imprint of ABC-CLIO, LLC

ABC-CLIO, LLC
130 Cremona Drive, P.O. Box 1911
Santa Barbara, California 93116-1911

This book is printed on acid-free paper (∞)

Manufactured in the United States of America

# Contents

# Preface

Those who do not remember the past are condemned to repeat it.

*George Santayana*

## WHO SHOULD READ THIS BOOK?

This book was written so that anyone with an interest in health inequity would be able to get something out of the discussion. Each chapter is designed to be an independent topic. There is no requirement that they be read in a sequence. If the reader is an advocate and wants to know more about lobbyists and health disparities, you can go straight to that chapter. If the reader is intrigued by the notion that fraud plays a role in health care inequity, you can go straight to that chapter. Readers with an interest in Medicaid will want to read the chapter on the topic and the chapter on young adults. Readers who want to think more about the history of health reform and disparities should start with the overview in chapter 1. Readers with an interest in disparities and financing will enjoy the discussion of business that has chosen health disparity populations as a niche market. Every chapter contains references to relevant legislative history. For scholars or anyone else, there is an index designed to facilitate identification of topics, people, and locations mentioned throughout the text.

# Acknowledgments

The opinions expressed in this text are strictly my own. I am ultimately responsible for any and all statements, facts, and conjectures. Any questions or comments should be directed to me. I would like to thank all the folks who read earlier draft versions of the chapters. Your feedback was invaluable. Thank you Kristen Blackwood, Robin Newton, Jeffrey Roberts, Robert Hudson, Sarah Frey, Phuong Trahn-Huynh, Geoffrey Elmore, Amy McKay, and others. I also want to thank Jessica Miles for developing my EndNote file. The extensive research included in this text would not be possible without this marvelous software. Special thanks to my two proof readers, Mary Boyd and A. W. Miles. Thanks to my new staff at the Institute of Gerontology. Without their patience and support, I would not have been able to bring this text to completion. I apologize for anyone who should have been named but was missed. Finally, I'd like to give a shout out to the Baucus Health Team—especially my homies in the bull pen. I learned so much from you guys!

# Introduction: How to Approach the Problem of Health Disparities and Health Care Reform

## THE DREAM RESEARCH PROJECT

Patient Protection and Affordable Care Act—P.L. 111–148 (hereafter referred to as ACA) was signed into law in March 2010. As every student of history knows, signing a law is just the beginning. Putting the law into practice is when its real impact happens. For researchers, this event creates a unique opportunity to study human behavior on a societal level. Currently, everything we know about disparities is studied after the fact using an historical perspective. The classic example is the Tuskegee Syphilis Study of African American World War I veterans, started in the 1930s. The idea was to monitor a group of infected veterans. The researchers already knew that late-stage syphilis was associated with complications. Medical researchers believed that although syphilis caused neurological and cardiac disease among European whites, the disease was harmless for blacks—an opinion held by many high-level medical professionals because of the widespread belief that whites and blacks were not the same. At the 1915 American Public Health Association meetings, papers showing syphilis-related deaths and stillbirths among African Americans were discussed. One demographer predicted that by 1960, the black population in the United States would die off because of syphilis. Clearly, that prediction was wrong. Inertia and racism kept the Tuskegee project active until 1972.

We can examine the motivations of these researchers and health care providers only through retrospective analyses. What if we could position ourselves at the beginning of the syphilis epidemic? Such would have been a dream research project. What would we learn about health care providers and their approach to black patients that we need to know now? How can those insights help in the implementation of this new legislation?

## FANTASY HEALTH DISPARITIES AND REFORM STUDY: WHO IS THE FOCUS OF OUR RESEARCH?

Our fantasy health disparities and reform project could track the experience of health care providers as the United States works to reform our health care system. Provider is a broad term that extends beyond physicians. Providers are hospitals, pharmaceutical companies, and equipment manufacturers. Any business that sells a service or product is a health care provider. Providers are on the frontlines, but everyone working in health care will be touched by some aspect of the change—and that means a lot of people. In 2009, about 9 percent of the total employed persons in the United States were employed in health care. On October 7, 2011, the Bureau of Labor Statistics reported that health care employment continued to expand, with an increase of 44,000 jobs in September 2011 alone. Within the industry, more than 26,000 jobs were created in ambulatory health care services, and more than 13,000 jobs were created in hospitals. Health care is one-sixth of the U.S. economy.

In the current climate of high unemployment and joblessness, change is terrifying. This is especially true for providers. To quote George Halvorson, CEO of Kaiser: "everyone else has a good business model that's working for them. There are two and a half trillion dollars in this market. There's no reason, if you have a comfortable cash flow, why would you do hard things and heavy lifting to get to a different model?"

The stakes are high in this period of implementation for everyone involved in health care, whether they are patients or direct consumers, medical doctors or nurses, pharmacists, medical technicians, researchers, or other staff at hospitals or clinics, pharmaceutical corporations, and health care insurance companies. Our fantasy researcher would have no shortage of subjects to follow in an on-the-ground study of human behavior.

## FANTASY HEALTH DISPARITIES AND REFORM STUDY: FRAME OF REFERENCE TO MEASURE CHANGE WHEN THERE IS CONSENSUS

The best study designs use an idea to provide a frame of reference. Scientists use the shape of the frame to articulate *what* will be measured and *why* we are measuring it. In sociology, a frame of reference is a set of basic assumptions or standards that determines and sanctions behavior. There are many, many ways to frame behavioral change. For example, almost every month the scientific community publishes a paper about the problems of helping people to change their diet, exercise, and smoking habits. The challenge confronting anyone trying to make these changes can be framed by the biological effect of the habit. Each of these activities is accompanied by a reward system that is wired into your biology. Each and every episode of consumption is rewarded with a response that reinforces continued behavior. Your body has a mechanism for telling your brain that it wants the item. Eating fatty, salty snacks rewards your taste buds. There are areas of the brain that respond to these foods as if they were heroin or cocaine. During the show *No Reservations,* host Anthony Bourdain eats roasted pork, rolls his eyes, and smacks his lips. That gesture says it all. Lounging on the sofa—particularly after the meal—is a pure pleasure. After Thanksgiving dinner, Americans are always grateful for a comfortable couch in front of the television. Smoking is another one of those behaviors accompanied by a system of biologically based rewards. Scientists since the time of Sigmund Freud have known that changing a behavior linked to a strong reward system is difficult. Not impossible—just difficult. There are individual success stories of dietary change, adoption of effective exercise habits, and smoking cessation. When the cost of not changing becomes greater than the reward for maintaining the status quo, change happens. These same habits become changeable during the teachable moment. Every clinician knows that after a heart attack, it is easy for some people to be guided through the changes in diet, exercise, and smoking. The structure of ACA is designed to create an environment in which the rewards for change exceed the rewards associated with the status quo.

The history surrounding the treatment of racial and ethnic groups by the medical establishment in the United States is ugly. It is easy to conduct painful and complex research when you are convinced that the being you are using in the experiment is less than human. However, over time, biomedical researchers have developed a system of research ethics, a system grounded in the belief that all human beings deserve our care and concern. This was a difficult process. In the past, there were significant social and economic rewards for conducting medical research without regard to the participant's well-being, such as happened in the Tuskegee Study. Medical researchers now work in the shadow of Nuremberg and other World War II–era crimes, from which arose better understandings of the nature of our fellow human beings and better standards for conducting research.

These standards protect study participants, and there are strong negative sanctions for those who violate those standards. For the medical community, this is behavioral change on a grand scale. Most of the changes have been in place only since the 1970s, but we need to understand them in order to evaluate ACA and its potential influence on patterns of inequity in the United States. The systemic changes that will result from the implementation of ACA will be similar in scale to the scope of change that occurred in the conduct of human subject research over the past 65 years.

This introduction is an opportunity for a prospective look at the impact of ACA on health care inequity. We will not know its impact on disparities, the product of inequity, for some time to come. We can, however, watch the changes in the behaviors of health care professionals. The following text reflects my fantasy for this study.

In this fantasy, we monitor the rollout of the Affordable Care Act (ACA). We could frame its challenge to the U.S. health care community as a behavior change problem. Just as changing the habits of diet, exercise, and smoking are tough, changing the behaviors of components within the health care industry is difficult. Not impossible, but difficult. As it is with changing any habitual behaviors, it will take a strong incentive to force change in the health care industry. In the ACA, that incentive is payment reform.

We could use any of a number of approaches to study behavioral change. I have two favorites. One approach assumes that an individual, an organization, or a region wants to change. They just do not know how to do it. This assumption makes the design of a study easy. Successful businesses do it all the time. Well-run organizations prepare for change with a self-study. This analysis is designed to identify and analyze the *strengths* and *weaknesses* of the organization. It encourages the involved parties to identify the *opportunities* and *threats*. This is called a SWOT analysis. Everyone in the organization is on board with the idea that change is needed. Everyone responsible for the changes understands his or her role in the process. Everyone can see the benefits for making the change. When there is organizational consensus, the application of new behaviors is rapid and smooth. The impact of the change is readily apparent.

For example, an individual might decide to alter his or her diet by substituting one bowl of fiber-rich cereal for one bowl of ice cream. He or she will notice a difference in the performance of the gastrointestinal tract in a few days. By persisting in that behavior for a month, the individual will notice a weight loss of two to four pounds. This rapid and positive feedback reinforces the new behavior and makes it easier to continue.

In the real world, there are many examples of successful organizational behavior change built on a foundation of consensus. Consider the problem of health care–associated infections. Health care–associated infections are infections that patients get while receiving treatment for another condition in some type of health care facility. It is estimated that health care–associated infections account for almost two million infections in a year. These infections are the most common complication of hospital care. They add to the cost of health care—between 28 billion dollars and 33 billion dollars each year! To address this problem, the Agency for Healthcare Research and Quality has developed a Comprehensive Unit Based Safety Program, which integrates communication, teamwork, and leadership to create and support a harm-free patient care culture. It provides a structured strategic framework for safety improvement. Improvements begin and end at the unit level, which is where actual health care takes place. The program is flexible enough to tap into staff wisdom, encouraging the unit to develop solutions for locally occurring hazards that pose the greatest risks. The program draws from frontline providers who have the most knowledge about safety hazards and the means to lessen the severity of those hazards, and provides a mechanism to help defend against infection hazards. This scalable program can be implemented throughout an organization.

There are five steps in the Comprehensive Unit Based Safety Program that are designed to incorporate evolving science-based knowledge to support continuing improvement. The measure of progress is change in patient safety. Each step builds on previous work. Frontline providers have the tools, metrics, and framework that they need to tackle the challenge of quality improvement. Consensus is built on a foundation of the science of safety. Staff are encouraged to assess their workplace and its culture of patient safety. A senior hospital executive works with the unit to improve communications. The top leadership learns along with the staff. Tools such as checklists, communication forums for team members, handwashing protocols, and systems of monitoring for infections reinforce the changes by making them part of the day-to-day process of work.

There is growing evidence that hospital-associated infections decline when intensive care units, surgical suites, and other areas adopt such tools. Health care–acquired infection can happen to anyone, but when the incidence of infection declines, the health care professionals working in these units experience increased satisfaction with the performance of their duties, and patients are more satisfied with the care they receive. As a result, any disparities associated with processes leading to health care–acquired infections improve.

## FANTASY HEALTH DISPARITIES AND REFORM STUDY: FRAME OF REFERENCE TO MEASURE CHANGE WHEN THERE IS DISAGREEMENT

The ACA transforms the relationship between health care delivery and payments by increasing emphasis on *quality* care. The framers of this legislation intended to use evidence-based practice to increase the quality of health care regardless of race, ethnicity, primary language, gender, or disability. My fantasy project examines provider readiness to adopt evidence-based practices. In the British journal *Quality and Safety in Health Care*, Shekelle argued that the resistance of physicians to clinical governance will continue until they can see how a real program works operationally resulting in a measurable leap in quality. In this 2002 article, Dr. Shekelle was referring to the National Health Service. The sentiment is descriptive of some provider attitudes in the United States.

There are unintended consequences of provider resistance to ACA. If Senator Rand Paul (R-Kentucky, ophthalmologist) were still in daily clinical practice, would he oppose the implementation of practice changes associated with ACA? What about Senator Tom Coburn (R-Oklahoma, family practice) or Senator John Barrasso (R-Wyoming, surgeon)? If these doctors were in daily medical practice, how would they respond to the quality improvement changes associated with ACA? Has anyone asked them about health care inequity in their states? Do they think about the unintended consequences of resistance to ACA's implementation? These are highly charged, political questions. That is not the purpose of the fantasy study. Rather, the goal is to measure the readiness to adopt the quality improvement processes presented in ACA and the association between stage of change and health care inequity.

Readiness to change is a concept commonly applied to diet, exercise, and smoking behaviors. Some individuals have never thought about changing or do not feel the need to do so. Others think about changing but do nothing about it. A third group tries to make the change but proceeds in fits and starts. A final group has successfully adopted a good diet and regular exercise and quit smoking and is, somehow, able to maintain the new behavior. These categories are associated with the Stage of Change Model as described by Prohaska and DiClemente. Is provider readiness to change practice an important but not well-measured social determinant of health care inequity? Although the 2008 presidential election represents a significant milestone in U.S. history, racism, classicism, gender bias, and xenophobia persist. Health care providers are human beings first. Before we got our professional training, we all grew up in our local communities. Nothing in our training is explicitly designed to confront our own biases. Some of us believe that we have no biases. Does missing insight into one's own beliefs create paths to inequity in health care delivery for one's patients? Does this personal blind spot create access barriers for a broad spectrum of disadvantaged groups? My dream study frames *provider attitudes* as a stage-of-change problem. If this study were done, we could use the results to design interventions that diminish the observed mistreatment, neglect, and scientific racism in health care. Although many hope that health care reform will address inequity, a formal study could measure the attitudes that may be linked to illness and death.

Imagine the four stages: "I don't need to change" (pre-contemplation); "Maybe I need to change" (contemplation); "I am trying this new strategy" (implementation); and "Wow, this change works" (maintenance). What would each say about the need for Cultural and Linguistically Appropriate Standards (CLAS) in health care? A pre-contemplation stage provider might make the argument that if the patient learned English, all of their problems would be solved. A contemplation stage provider might make the argument that CLAS is a good idea, but it costs too much. An implementation stage provider might say that he or she is trying to learn medical Spanish, but everyone laughs when he or she speaks. Finally, the maintenance stage provider has hired staff for the office who speak Spanish. Her patient base in the local Latino community is growing. What would the Healthcare Effectiveness Data and Information Set statistics for each provider look like? The pre-contemplation and contemplation stage provider might have a lower proportion of patients with up-to-date immunizations, screenings, and poorly controlled chronic conditions. The barrier for their patients is communication with the office. At these two early stages, providers might be inclined to attribute the missing preventive services to health illiteracy, willful noncompliance, or mistrust of the health care system. Help the provider advance a stage or two and perhaps patient outcomes will improve.

As director of a hospital, how could I use this stage of readiness measurement to implement change across providers? Measuring readiness to adopt CLAS could influence my institution's Consumer Assessment of Healthcare Providers and Systems (CAHPS) scores. One item in particular asks, "During this hospital stay, how often did doctors treat you with courtesy and respect?" When the providers are arranged by stage of readiness to change, which stage would have the highest proportion rated as *usually* or *always*? Which ones are more likely to be rated as *sometimes* or *never*?

Because this is a fantasy research project, we do not know the answers to these questions. The design of this project would have to be useful in creating a series of changes targeting correctable disparities. What about CAHPS rating averages of providers who serve patients with low literacy or low income? The opportunity created by ACA for a prospective study of changes in health disparities is a golden opportunity. Findings from this fantasy study can be applied to the larger universe of patients and providers because Medicare rules and regulations in the United States are typically adopted by private insurers, Medicaid, and the Veterans Health Administration (VHA).

There is a gain for providers who participate in this fantasy project. The Tax Relief and Health Care Act of 2006 established the Physician Quality Reporting Initiative. It is housed within the Centers for Medicare and Medicaid Services. Among other features, it includes an incentive payment for eligible professionals who satisfactorily report data on quality measures for services provided to Medicare beneficiaries. A part of the ACA beginning in 2011 gives physicians the opportunity to earn an additional half percent of Medicare Part B billing by working with a Maintenance of Certification (MOC) entity. The Stages of Change framework of this fantasy study has the potential for becoming a program practice assessment. Successfully completing a qualified practice assessment is one path to obtaining the incentive payment. In lay language, this means Medicare could potentially pay a bonus to providers who participate in the fantasy project. Aside from the Physician Quality Reporting Initiative, there is additional benefit to providers with a large number of patients with public insurance plans like Medicare and Medicaid. Their comments are invaluable and necessary if we are to make improvements in ACA policy.

The critical period for measuring ACA's impact on access barriers is now slightly more than 12 months from ACA's becoming a law. Barring any action in the Supreme Court, ACA should be fully implemented by 2014. Interviewing providers during the next five years would allow researchers to link provider stage of change with the uptake of quality improvement policies and, in turn, future reductions in health care inequity.

However, we are already seeing changes to the implementation of ACA. One casualty is the long-term care portion of the legislation. The Community Living Assistance Services and Supports Act has just been dropped because of federal budgetary concerns. What does the retreat on long-term care mean for future cohorts of impoverished elders? Currently, impoverished persons who require long-term care are dependent on state Medicaid programs. These programs are under budgetary duress. Will we see a return to the conditions observed among frail elders in the period before Medicaid was enacted? Will we see large numbers of impoverished elders living in the community with unmet home care needs? Unmet long-term care needs for frail elders will become an age-based disparity if present trends continue. The process of meeting those needs could be defined as a correctable disparity. Understanding attitudinal resistance would improve the structure of long-term care policy.

In the fantasy project, we can array providers by their Medicare experience. Some have much more than others. What is the relationship between experience with public insurance programs, policy implementation, and stage of change? Medicare, with its near universal coverage, provides an unbiased sample of patients from diverse backgrounds. Is stage of change linked to patient diversity? The Medicare population includes a large proportion of persons experiencing health disparities. Some are younger enrollees in the End Stage Renal Disease Program, as well as low-income elders who are dually eligible for both Medicare and Medicaid. In addition, the Medicare population includes the Medicare Advantage subscribers— a largely white, well-educated, and highly resourced group of elders. By emphasizing Medicare participants, our universe of provider recruits can be quantified by their professional association to this population. We can recruit physicians, nurses, social workers, and other health care professionals—a mix that is more diverse than is usually represented in provider studies. Medicare beneficiaries are most likely to require the services of a broad array of health care professionals.

The Stage of Change Model provides clues that mark predictable stages. Providers are ultimately the final arbiter of their own practice. It is important, however, that we test the notion that provider adoption of evidence-based practice proceeds through predictable stages. The changes in health care delivery mandated in health reform are not simple. These changes will require time to implement. Other studies of behavioral change indicate that movement to the next stage is preceded by a consideration of the pros and cons associated with making a change.

Health care providers—like everyone else—base some of their opinions on reports from public media. This means that providers can be diverse in their political views of the new policies. The fantasy project will need design innovations to accommodate this complexity. Perhaps we can assess provider politics through a triangulation process—employ multiple methods to capture a provider's true feelings. Most people would be frightened by the idea that a provider is biased against their group. Providers might be ashamed to admit the bias. By using multiple methods to study the same topic, we will achieve a deeper understanding of behavioral change in health care delivery.

There a number of advantages associated with this fantasy study. We could accurately identify factors that influence the opinions of health care professionals as real events happen. As much as we might try, using historical data does not accurately capture influences and behaviors. Actions and motivations are always distorted by the lens of present-day sensibilities. There are modern studies of physician attitudes concerning practice change. Most of those studies ask study subjects to *imagine change*. Sometimes, imagining a thing is far more satisfying than actually experiencing it. This is not logical, but it is often true. The same can be said for changes in health care practices. The fantasy study is useful for keeping a record of the introduction of *quality* measures into the U.S. health care delivery system. Public health history is full of instances of process change: the introduction of vital statistics, changes in childbirth practices, and outlawing public spitting. All of these changes have led to improved public health. No one really knows about the resistance that had to be overcome to achieve these changes. Right now, we do not have a clear road map for implementation of ACA. It is a lot like making a cake. Put the ingredients together in the wrong sequence, and you have a mess. Sugar and butter go first. Next, you add the flour. Finally, you add eggs and milk or water. Follow the sequence, and you have a delicious cake. Does provider *readiness* to change practice have a direct impact on health care inequity? If our fantasy study confirms that idea, we can use the information to restructure the educational experience of providers as they begin their training. We can reframe the model of behavioral change to include modifiable attitudes of health care professionals. Rather than hopelessness around health disparities, they become correctable issues.

Can the new health care reform act—the Patient Protection and Affordable Care Act of 2010 (ACA)—diminish health disparities in the United States? The ACA is a consumer-focused, market-based legislation. Most sections are not expressed in an explicit race- or ethnic-focused language. Will this market-based approach change our concept of health disparities? This book explores the potential of this consumer-protection approach to diminish health disparities. In the United States, almost 200 million persons obtain health insurance from their employers. Do these plans create health care inequity? Regulating the private insurance market is a core policy of the ACA. What does the ACA mean to public plans such as Medicaid? Some say that Medicaid creates health care inequity. Chapter 2 presents a detailed analysis of Medicaid and its role in the large picture of health care inequity. Is poor quality care part of the disparities puzzle? Chapter 3 explores the ACA approach to improving the quality and efficiency of health care. This is the most complex portion of the new law. It is not widely discussed in media coverage. Improving health in the United States will require behavioral change by both patients and health care professionals. If quality is an issue, what types of attitudes and behaviors do health care professionals need to change?

Does disparity evolve out of the way we do business? Chapter 4 describes six businesses whose mission involves providing care or insurance to Medicaid beneficiaries. What do their chief executive officers say about health disparities? Health care is one-sixth of the U.S. economy. Lower costs are a two-edged sword: good for persons who purchase care, not so good for persons who make a living selling health care services and commodities. What, if anything, will ACA regulations do to change the practices of these niche companies? What do these models teach us about the safety net hospital system? Safety net hospitals started during a time when illness in the United States was dominated by epidemics of infectious diseases and a demographically young population. Our current illness pattern is dominated by chronic disease in an older population. Business models designed to care for chronic disease are very different from the safety net model of hospital-centered care. Will ACA improve stability of the safety net system? Does the law provide the resources for safety net hospitals to make needed changes? Policy has the potential to make things both better and worse.

The ACA debate was characterized by commentary from almost all sectors of America. Did any group explicitly lobby for policy to end health disparities? Chapter 5 explores this question. What would advocacy for policies to end health disparities look like? Is the policy request generic? A generic advocate might say "Health care for all!" Is the request specific? A specific request might be "Free health care for all children under the age of 5 years." A portion of the chapter distinguishes between lobbying and advocacy. There is historical precedence for advocacy at the federal level dating back to the early 1900s. Two groups in particular—the March of Dimes and the American Cancer Society—have been particularly successful. Why does the March of Dimes continue to be so successful in their efforts on behalf of mothers and children? The earliest health equity advocacy evolved out of efforts to overcome cancer. The history of this advocacy by the American Cancer Society is placed within the context of ACA development.

There are two other specialty chapters on health care fraud and the needs of young adults. What about health care fraud? During the writing of ACA, fraud and its contribution to the cost of health care was a topic for debate. ACA reflects this debate. Does the design of our payment system encourage fraud? News reports and legal cases provide evidence of fraud in public programs. Are there similar levels of fraud in private plans? Chapter 6 discusses fraud, its potential role in health disparities, and the ACA approach. In chapter 7 the plight of young adults as they begin this phase of life is placed in the spotlight. ACA Title I and II contain policies that anticipate the loss of health insurance associated with the transitions of young adulthood. The barriers to health care faced by young adults with disabilities are examined. What does ACA do for this demographic group? The development of Medicare solved barriers to hospital care experienced by older adults and African Americans. Does ACA solve the barriers to care experienced by young adults? Finally, the topic of correctable disparities will be visited in chapter 8.

Each chapter in this work is supported by references from court cases, historical documents, research reports, and media stories. Together, this book broadens our view of U.S. health care inequity—its causes and solutions.

## BIBLIOGRAPHY

Shekelle, P. G. "Why Don't Physicians Enthusiastically Suggest Quality Improvement Programmes?" *Quality and Safety in Health Care* 11, no. 6 (2002), doi:10.1136/ahc.11.1.6.

# CHAPTER 1

## Overview: Diminishing Health Disparities

Though we are all consumers in an insurance model of health care delivery, the term *consumer* is not synonymous with *patient*. Employers who purchase insurance for their workforce are also consumers. In the United States, consumers repeatedly express two fundamental concerns: *Will I get the care I need, when I need it?* Inability to access timely, safe, and effective health care is linked to health disparities. *How much will it cost?* This question is a concern for both patients and employers. Each chapter returns to this core question: Will policies that have a consumer basis facilitate quality access?

ACA policy is less like the Civil Rights Act and more like Roosevelt's New Deal. The last major health care legislation—Medicare—emerged out of the civil rights movement as a social medical insurance program. Its emphasis on civil rights reflects deliberate planning by policy makers. Health care inequity and policy-based remedies have historic roots in the United States. Before 1964, sick elders were not treated in the hospital. The civil rights of older adults and their access to health care were improved with the enactment of Medicare. In 1964, older Americans did not have employer-sponsored health insurance after retirement. Medicare was a remedy for this age-based health care inequity. In 1964, the high cost of hospital-based care for elders was given as the justification for limiting access. With Medicare, for the first time, there was guaranteed hospital care. Medicare also served a civil rights agenda. To receive Medicare payments, hospitals were required to accept *all* patients regardless of race. With financing as a tool, Medicare also forced the racial integration of hospitals in the South. Medicare continued a process of desegregation in hospitals, which began with the Hill Burton Hospital Survey and Construction Act of 1946 (Hill Burton) (Public Law 79-725). Hill Burton provided funds to upgrade hospitals in communities across the United States. To obtain these funds, public hospitals were obligated to open their doors to everyone. Hill Burton funds supported the building of hospitals such as Cook County Hospital in Chicago and Charity Hospital in New Orleans. The framers of both Medicare and Hill Burton understood that placement of federal dollars was a key strategy to decreasing barriers to hospital-based health care.

New Deal programs like Social Security provide financial resources for households. ACA Title I, Subtitle A, Part A, reforms the private health insurance marketplace. This title benefits the 200 million Americans whose households obtain their health care resources from the workplace. The Social Security Act is not concerned with civil rights. In fact, farmers, domestics, and sharecroppers were specifically excluded when Social Security was enacted in 1935. In the southern states, large numbers of blacks were engaged in these occupations. In the northern states, domestics were mostly immigrants from Europe. The omission of these groups created income inequity by limiting eligibility for these occupational groups when they were too old to work. Does the ACA create inequity between types of employer-sponsored health care plans? The answer to this larger question is evolving as the law is being implemented. It is clear that the ACA creates stability in private insurance plans by establishing rules for coverage where none existed. Before the ACA, the private insurance markets— where individuals and employers purchase coverage—had no ground rules establishing the essential benefits and no rules defining the conduct of the health insurance business. Just as Social Security became the prototype for retirement plans, the ACA specifies a framework for health insurance plans.

When we speak of health care broadly, it is important to remember that *health care inequity* and *health disparities* are not synonymous terms. *Inequity* is a process. *Disparity* is a byproduct of prolonged inequity. Policy creates processes. More than 50 years of academic studies link race, household reserves, and other characteristics of the patient with health disparity. Does ACA policy acknowledge this body of research? If health care inequity is a racial issue, does ACA policy focus on specific racial groups? The ACA has explicitly introduced the collection of data on race, ethnicity, language, and disability of the patient as a requirement for payment by public plans. If health care inequity is an economic issue, do we see a policy addressing the needs of low-wage workers? The ACA has several policies for low-wage workers. If health care inequity is an issue of gender or age discrimination, do we see a policy that targets women or older adults? Before the ACA, companies routinely charged higher premiums for women and older adults. There were no guidelines for this pricing structure. Both individuals and communities were disadvantaged by this practice. Workers living in communities with higher proportions of older adults and women also paid higher premiums for their employer-sponsored health insurance plans. Individuals were disadvantaged as they progressed through middle age since their insurance premiums increased exponentially. Middle-aged persons—particularly women—who wanted to start a small business found the cost of health insurance premiums to be unaffordable. Does the New Deal structure of the ACA create or diminish these health care inequities?

In the United States, almost all health care is financed through a third-party insurance company. This is the business model for all insurance plans—both public and private. Contracts are made with companies who, in turn, negotiate with health care providers. *Provider* is a broad term that extends beyond physicians. Providers are hospitals, pharmaceutical companies, and equipment manufacturers. Any business that sells a service or product is a health care provider. This definition of provider will become important in the later chapters on fraud, lobbying, and business models. By coordinating the financial transactions between providers, insurance companies play a complex role in the U.S. health care system. Most insurance companies are privately held, but there are nonprofit companies in the mix. These companies provide a service to individuals and their employers and also a profit for their shareholders. Some insurance companies provide their services to state Medicaid plans. In chapter 4, we examine the business models of AmeriHealth Mercy, Molina Healthcare, and Centene Corporation. The states contract with specialty insurance companies to manage the health care benefits for their Medicaid beneficiaries. Yes, there are private companies in the business of managing public health care plans. Only a few state governments manage their own Medicaid plans. In chapter 2, I discuss the Oklahoma history during the 1990s with managed Medicaid and its evolution to a state-managed plan.

Medicaid covers every aspect of health care—prenatal care and delivery, emergency care, hospitalization, and long-term care for disabled persons. It is as close as we can get in the United States to cradle-to-grave coverage. Medicaid is financed using the resources of individual states with federal matching dollars. Medicaid is not the only public health insurance plan. Medicare is the largest insurance company in the world with almost 100 million beneficiaries. Medicare finances health care by combining beneficiary premiums with tax dollars to pay providers. Providers, in turn, pay personnel, build health care facilities, and oversee the goods that are used for treatment. Unlike Medicaid, Medicare does not provide maternity care or support for long-term care in institutions. Medicare is focused on chronic-disease care—outpatient, hospital, medical equipment, and medications. These are the most profitable segments of the health care industry. Maternity care is less profitable. This distinction between the cost of Medicaid maternal and child health services and Medicare chronic care was made in a letter to the speaker of the House from the Congressional Budget Office (March 2010). The Congressional Budget Office (CBO) provided estimates for the period 2010 through 2019 for two subtitles of ACA. During this period, *Subtitle L: Maternal and child health* had a total estimated cost of two billion dollars. The CBO estimated that 42 billion dollars were required to fill Part D—coverage gap in the Medicare donut hole. With the exception of newly emergent long-term acute-care hospitals, the long-term custodial care is also less profitable. At each point in the discussion of health disparities, consideration must be given to the role of public plans and the corporate structure of health care delivery in the United States. How big does a public plan need to be to run a cost-efficient model of health care delivery?

The only real exception to the third-party management strategy in the United States is the Veterans Health Administration (VHA) system. The VHA owns the location and structure of its clinics and hospitals. The VHA also negotiates over medication prices. Almost all physicians in the VHA system are salaried. The VHA has an electronic health care record system that has been in place since the mid-1980s. In the early 1990s, the VHA had a reputation for delivering limited, poor-quality care. Patient dissatisfaction with health care drove its own internal health care reform process. By 2000, the VHA showed substantial improvement in overall performance and patient satisfaction. At present, it is the most highly rated health care system in the United States. What about costs? Getting an estimate of the cost of care in the VHA is complex because the dollars are divided across a number of categories. It supports medical education by paying the salaries of teaching physicians as well as providing training sites for the health care workforce. Almost 40 percent of U.S. medical school faculty is paid by the VHA. The VHA, therefore, plays a major role in U.S. medical education. It pays for facilities. Other costs in the VHA go to employee wages and benefits. Finally, the VHA operates a research and development component through its Veterans Administration Office of Research and Development. The per capita cost of VHA reflects all of these missions.

Like the rest of the United States, the VHA patient base is aging. Older patients require more care. During the same period of quality improvement, the VHA added new long-term care services for these aging World War II and later veterans. Part of the improved patient satisfaction is directly linked to the VHA's commitment to provide these services to veterans living in the community, which is one strategy that lowers the overall cost of health care. Greater numbers needing this care, however, have the opposite effect on budgets. As the veterans from Iraq and Afghanistan return, many will require the comprehensive medical care delivered by the VHA. These veterans will drive the costs associated with immediate and long-term care. The cost for supporting the VHA is an evolving story. The U.S. health care system is traveling a parallel course.

Does health care inequity exist in the VHA? In the current system, the answer to this question is not clear. There is evidence of differences based on race and ethnicity in outcomes when comparing black and white veterans. While standardized procedures have led to smaller racial disparities, there is residual disparity attributable to clinical judgment. Black veterans are less likely to use surgical procedures. Whether this is a choice of the veterans or a systematic bias in the system is not known at this time. The main lesson from the VHA experience is that attention to consumer satisfaction can diminish some aspects of health care inequity but not all of it. Within the VHA, quality-improvement programs continue the drive to diminish disparity. As will be explained in chapter 3, quality is not just a generic term. It is a set of procedures designed to achieve health care that is safe, effective, patient-centered, timely, and equitable. The VHA is a delivery system committed to quality care. In 2009, the VHA's Clinical Research Pharmacy Coordinating Center in Albuquerque, New Mexico, received a Malcolm Baldrige National Quality Award. The Baldrige Award is named after a former U.S. secretary of commerce, Malcolm Baldrige. Secretary Baldrige was an advocate for the idea that quality management was the key to prosperity and sustainability in all businesses. Winning a Baldrige Award is an arduous process. Many of the quality initiatives in ACA Title III were developed first in the VHA. The nonprofit organization National Quality Forum is one of the groups that are working on improving the quality of U.S. health care. National Quality Forum has been around since the 1990s. It is clear that quality reduces race-based gaps in health care within the VHA. Will quality initiatives have a similar impact on the larger U.S. health care system? National Quality Forum is working to translate VHA lessons into broader practices.

VHA improvements were achieved with an increasing emphasis on patient satisfaction. Measuring satisfaction requires a patient-centered approach to care. The ACA uses a patient-centered language to develop a consumer point of view. By incorporating the consumer's voice into the payment process, the ACA reforms health care payment policy. One example is the *Hospital Value Based Purchasing Program* (Title III, Section 3001). This section mandates that data from the Hospital Consumer Assessment of Healthcare Providers and Systems survey be used to reward quality with incentive payments. Items in the survey ask patients to rate their in-hospital patient experience communicating with nurses, doctors, and staff. Hospital payments are linked to patient rating on these items. Incorporating the voice of the consumer is a new policy in the structure of health care payments. This book takes a similar approach. To incorporate the views of involved groups, there are direct quotes throughout this book. These quotes are taken from publically available sources. They represent individuals with a direct experience of a barrier in health care. In many cases, these individuals are usually excluded from the policy discussion. Instead, their views are represented by advocates. Advocates have always understood the power of personal testimony. Consumer ratings in these surveys can be used by local advocates to lower health disparities. The results of these surveys are available at www.hospitalcompare.hhs. gov. Individual hospital ratings are available on this website. Patients and advocates can use these data to communicate directly with area hospital boards. Through the availability of surveys, the ACA provides data to local consumer advocacy groups. In short, the ACA policy increases the linkage between consumer satisfaction and payment.

Employers are also consumers of health care. While cost is an issue for them, there are other concerns. Business Roundtable and the U.S. Chamber of Commerce (the Chamber) are two advocates for the concerns of chief executive officers and other business leaders. Each has advocated for access to Medicare claims data. Why? Employers who purchase health insurance cannot track the performance of physicians, pharmacies, and hospitals providing care to their employees. Employers cannot reward high-performing health care. They cannot detect fraudulent charges for service. If a single pharmacy charges excessive rates for the employees of an individual business, there is no way to *see* it. Even the largest employer-sponsored plans cannot detect this kind of problem. Why? The number of individual employees using a singular pharmacy is small. Businesses with multiple operations across the United States have the same problem with measurement that a small business operating in one place has. Detecting poor quality service or outright fraud is only possible with a very large pool of beneficiaries. Medicare claims data, which come from more than 100 million beneficiaries, meet the size requirements needed to measure service and detect fraud. The ACA contains new requirements for Medicare data-sharing rules. In August 2011, Business Roundtable and the Chamber gave written comments to the Centers for Medicare and Medicaid Services describing the structure of their data needs. Maria Ghazal of the Business Roundtable specifically mentions the stringent patient privacy protections that should be in place during data sharing. Randel Johnson and Kate Mahoney of the Chamber of Commerce emphasize the elimination of proprietary elements from prescription drug data before sharing. Both organizations emphasize that price and performance evaluation is the rationale for access to these claims data. Employers are consumers of health care through their purchase of employee insurance. Businesses are accustomed to analyzing cost drivers for their operations. Health care is one of those areas that have not been open to this type of scrutiny. The ACA, through its rules defining a process for making Medicare data available, aims to improve the performance of health care in employer-sponsored plans.

Most Americans, at one time or another in their lives, encounter a barrier that slows health care access. These barriers are most likely to appear at predictable points in the life cycle—birth, transition to young adult independence, transitions between jobs, transition to retirement, and dependency in old age. In the United States, transition-related barriers are associated with coverage issues. If you do not have employer-based insurance or a policy you purchased for yourself, your next possible option is a public insurance plan. Medicaid and Medicare are public plans. Not everyone is eligible to participate in these plans. Health insurance can be thought of as a surrogate for a credit card. The more benefits in your plan, the higher its value. Comprehensive insurance is equivalent to having a platinum credit card. If you have it, any health care provider will be happy to serve your needs. The vendors know that they will be paid promptly. On the other end of the health insurance spectrum is Medicaid. In the view of providers (doctors, hospitals, clinics), Medicaid is a debit card. Payment is slow and involves an enormous hassle. Many providers refuse this card. Across the United States, Medicaid goes by many names—Passport (Kentucky), Tenn Care (Tennessee), and others. Rebranding does not remove its stigma from the mind of a vendor. In chapter 2, I discuss the details of

Medicaid and its provider issues. Providers' perception of Medicaid creates barriers to health care.

Race, ethnicity, or primary language can create barriers to health care. Public hospitals have an historical role in open-access health care. Public hospitals serve multiple purposes in our health care delivery system by training physicians and providing a culturally comfortable environment for patients. These hospitals are most likely to provide care to persons without health insurance as well as those with public insurance plans. With this client base, public hospitals are starved for the resources to make needed capital investments. Without capital investment, it is difficult to support quality-improvement programs of the hospital. Does the ACA provide the resources required by these institutions for capital investment? There are business models that suggest that quality improvement leads to smaller differences between black and white death rates. The ACA also provides more resources for historically black colleges and universities. The graduates of Howard University, Meharry Medical College, and Morehouse School of Medicine have the highest rates of physicians who choose to serve these communities after graduation. Without these institutions, there would be fewer physicians in these areas. Prior to the enactment of the ACA, John Iglehart wrote an essay outlining changes in medical education financing that would promote the model used by these historically black colleges and universities and increase the numbers of primary care physicians. The Council on Graduate Medical Education, in its 2010 report, argued that the ACA did not go far enough in its financial support of safety net institutions. Some of the provisions in the ACA increase resources to institutions with a primary mission of service. Some of the provisions in the ACA, like disproportionate share payments to hospitals, decrease this source of funds. In short, the ACA is not designed to provide resources for capital improvements. Byrd and Clayton provide ample documentation for a history of segregated care and training in their definitive study of race, history, and U.S. health care. Historically, insufficient infrastructure has had deadly consequences for racial and ethnic groups in the U.S. health care system. Studies show that these risks persisted in 2010. This is particularly true for persons who do not communicate in English. Many patients who use English as a second language are legal citizens. They were actively recruited to fulfill U.S. workforce needs. These workers suffer from both language-based and race- and ethnicity-based barriers. With the *National Cultural and Language Standards,* the need for appropriate language services was identified as a component of quality health care. This standard recognizes the millions of patients served by U.S. hospitals.

Only 19 percent of U.S. hospitals currently meet the mandated standards for language-appropriate care. Communication barriers also contribute to higher rates of postsurgical complications for all persons who use English as a secondary language.

What about persons with Medicaid coverage? If asked, what would they say about health care inequity? If you wanted to speak with these consumers, you could visit a Federally Qualified Health Center (FQHC). These centers are nonprofit private or public entities designated to serve medically underserved populations and areas, migrant and seasonal farm workers, the homeless, or residents of public housing. These centers exist in U.S. statute. FQHCs are required by law to provide comprehensive outpatient health care. This includes hospital access for their patients who need it. To receive federal funds, FQHCs must adhere to quality standards of medical care. If you walked into the lobby of an FQHC and struck up a conversation with people waiting to be seen, what would you hear about inequity and reform? Would anyone understand the idea of disparities? FQHCs are the only nonmilitary health care facilities in the United States open to the public *regardless of the ability to pay*. It is as close to a Canadian-style health service or a British-style national system as we can get. FQHC clients generally have public insurance plans. More than 38 percent of their clients are uninsured, and 47 percent receive insurance through public plans such as Medicaid and Medicare. Approximately 15 percent of the patients seeking care at FQHCs have private insurance. These individuals have employer plans with limited benefits and high deductibles. In 2009, there were 19 million persons served by FQHCs across the United States.

Each FQHC is an independent site for care. There is no connectivity between locations. FQHCs employ more than 123,000 persons across the United States. In communities with high rates of unemployment, FQHCs can be a source of employment close to home. There are collaborative networks of FQHCs that engage in self-study to improve health care delivery. These practice-based research networks can be found in California and across the Southeast. FQHCs have limited capital investment available to improve their infrastructure. In addition to payments from insurance, they obtain some of their financing by competing for research funding. These research funds come from agencies such as the Centers for Disease Control and Prevention, the Agency for Healthcare Research and Quality, and the Bureau of Health Professions. Unlike a private medical practice, the FQHC is governed by a board with mandated representation of its patients. For each FQHC, the board represents community demographics for race, ethnicity, and gender. A portion of the board must represent the service area community. These members are selected for their expertise in community affairs, local government, finance and banking, legal affairs, trade unions, and other commercial and industrial concerns, or they may be social service agencies within the community. FQHCs stabilize public health in the United States. This is a significant but untold story in U.S. health care delivery.

In most areas of the United States, FQHC clientele are folks with little or no health insurance. Some use English as a second language; many left school before completing the 12th grade. The racial, ethnic, and age composition of the group is highly dependent on the local geography. In south Texas, for example, you will find that many are natural-born U.S. citizens whose families have lived in segregated south Texas neighborhoods for generations. Many work in the tourism industry of Texas. Many of the tourism-related businesses do not offer health insurance. Employee wages are so low that many workers are eligible for Medicaid. This scenario is not unique to Texas; it exists wherever there are large numbers of service-industry jobs. If you are in the Woodlawn area of Chicago's South Side, you will see mostly those whose grandparents and great grandparents migrated out of the southern United States during the 1920s. Persons in this neighborhood are also highly likely to work for employers who offer health insurance plans with limited benefits. Maternity care and preventive services are generally not included in their employer-sponsored plans. These limited plans are analogous to *debit cards*. If you are in the Portland neighborhood of Louisville, Kentucky, you can interview whites whose relatives moved out of Appalachia years ago to work for industries that no longer exist. Louisville is a river town along the Ohio River and at one time had a diverse industrial base—manufacturing, meatpacking, and tobacco. Again, FQHC clients in Louisville work in low-wage jobs and have insurance with limited benefits. The Portland neighborhood does not have many alternatives for medical or dental care. The FQHC is the only provider of dental care for the entire west side of Louisville. The common thread linking FQHC waiting rooms in south Texas, Chicago, and Louisville is the simple fact that everyone is there to see a doctor.

By any criteria, the individuals who choose an FQHC for health care are consumers with debit cards. If we surveyed these FQHC consumers, what would they say about the quality and accessibility of their health care? Quality and consumer satisfaction are a critical component of the ACA. In fact, the ACA reforms payment policy by linking it to consumer satisfaction. Title III, in particular, is dedicated to improving care by incorporating the voice of the consumer. How would FQHC clients rate the communication that takes place with their doctors and nurses? How likely are they to recommend the facility to friends and family? In subsequent chapters, we will show data to answer these specific questions. This overview is focused on broader questions. Whose voice is heard in the national debate about health disparities? What do these voices say? Are the consumers in the FQHC waiting room heard? The debit card metaphor is one way to define their potential to experience disparity and link it to the insurance model of health care financing in the United States. This process creates barriers for some, but not all, health care consumers. Provider bias against consumers with less desirable insurance plans reinforces health care inequity.

Consumerism in health care is not a threat to providers who value their patients. After all, patients drive the demand for the goods and services. This concept is threatening when providers conclude that patients are incapable of acting responsibly in their self-interest and are unwilling to take an active role. As such providers might say, "Patients, who are incapable of acting responsibly, cannot be allowed to express dissatisfaction with care. *After all, they don't really know what's good for them.*" This notion is sometimes expressed by providers within the context of a health disparity discussion. This notion runs counter to the national discussion of consumerism in health care. Maximizing consumer choice and increasing consumer satisfaction were two sentiments expressed by both proponents and opponents of the ACA. In Deloitte's 2009 longitudinal survey of consumers, the highest rates of satisfaction with health plans were expressed by enrollees in Medicare (70%) and military health programs (67%). Persons who purchased an individual plan in the private markets were least satisfied (45%). Lisa Cooper-Patrick's (1999) studies of patient–physician communication show that participatory decision making is a component of satisfaction for all racial groups. All racial and ethnic groups prefer an active role in making decisions about medical care. Blanchard and Lurie (2004) found that when a patient reports feeling disrespected during treatment, this feeling can have a detrimental impact on health care outcomes. When patients identify race as the source of disrespect, they are less likely to get a routine physical exam, follow a doctor's advice, or receive appropriate secondary preventive care for diabetes, heart disease, and hypertension. We are all health care consumers, distinguished by the type of card we carry. It is common for a consumer to be treated differently by providers because of that card. After all, it is difficult to book a hotel with a debit card. However, in the context of health care, linking consumer disrespect to credit card type has deadly consequences. Card-type preference may be mistaken for racism. The consumerism basis of health care financing influences the behaviors of patients and providers. Consumerism also influences the political dialogue of inequity and disparity in health care access.

Politics shape policy. Many voices were heard during the debate leading up to enactment of the ACA. As this book progresses, you will hear those voices. In most cases, we report the actual words of the speaker. Preference will always be given to eyewitness reports rather than opinions. C-SPAN and YouTube archives of hearings create the opportunity for each of us to hear these voices. In the text, opinion is given priority if it comes from actual consumers or providers. These priority voices have surrogates on both the political left and right. The surrogates have their own political agenda, which sometimes bears no relationship to health care inequity. Sometimes, surrogate voices are difficult to distinguish from priority voices. Sometimes, it is clear that a surrogate voice is speaking. Surrogates emphasize outcome over experience. For example, when writing for the Center for American Progress, Lesley Russell speaks as a surrogate. She suggests that communities of color will derive a greater benefit from the ACA. The point here is not to dismiss the validity of her statement. There are excellent analyses supporting her view. Sometimes, however, the surrogate suggests a political perspective. For example, Klick and Satel at the American Enterprise Institute published a monograph promoting the idea that there is no role for physician behavior in the development of health disparities. These liberal and conservative views are grounded in different beliefs. What is the difference? Liberals value collective responsibility and public good. Conservatives value individual responsibility and choice. This grounding leads to very different health care reform policies. These values also create very different frames for inequity and disparity in health care access. In shaping the final law, considerable effort was made trying to create a policy that could accommodate these very different values. Sometimes, the values of the speaker are clear. Sometimes, they can only be inferred from the tone of the comment.

Politics cannot be divorced from policy. This is important to keep in mind because political positioning is used to drive action. Political opponents generated resistance to enacting the ACA during debate, with allegations ranging from *death panels* to *hidden taxes*. Political debates and the call for action or resistance are not new. There is historical evidence of presidential concern over this type of resistance. For example, President Lyndon B. Johnson directly confronted resistance to the Civil Rights Act of 1964. From the East Room of the White House on July 2, 1964, he made the following points:

> We must not approach the observance and enforcement of this law in a vengeful spirit. Its purpose is not to punish. Its purpose is not to divide, but to end divisions—divisions which have all lasted too long. Its purpose is national, not regional. . . . Its purpose is to promote a more abiding commitment to freedom, a more constant pursuit of justice, and a deeper respect for human dignity. . . . We will achieve these goals because most Americans are law abiding citizens who want to do what is right. . . . This is why the Civil Rights Act relies first on voluntary compliance, then on the efforts of local communities and states to secure the rights of citizens. It provides for the national authority to step in only when others cannot or will not do the job. . . . This Civil Rights Act is a challenge to all of us to go to work in our communities and our states, in our homes and in our hearts, to eliminate the last vestiges of injustice in our beloved country. . . . So tonight I urge every public official, every religious leader, every business and professional man, every workingman, every housewife—I urge every American—to join in this effort to bring justice and hope to all our people—and to bring peace to our land. . . . My fellow citizens, we have come now to a time of testing. We must not fail. Let us close the springs of racial poison. Let us pray for wise and understanding hearts. Let us lay aside irrelevant differences and make our nation whole.

In short, he makes an appeal to Americans across the political spectrum to work together to make this new law happen. This message is consistent with Johnson's larger Great Society framework of helping the less fortunate in the United States.

President Barack Obama addressed resistance to newly enacted legislation in a meeting on the six-month anniversary of the ACA enactment. U.S. Department of Health and Human Services (HHS) representatives and faith-based community leaders attended the conference call. The participants in the call were largely supporters of the law. The president was promoting neighbor-to-neighbor conversation to overcome resistance. If President Johnson had arranged this call, the attendees would have been drawn from the ranks of elected officials—not advocates and members of the executive branch of the federal government:

> I wanted to have this call because we've got a big day coming up—
> the six month anniversary of the passage of the Affordable Care
> Act. . . . When people better understand the ACA, they'll understand
> that, I think, this is not something being done to them, but something
> that is really going to be valuable [for] them. . . . The ACA is now
> law. So as—I think all of you can be really important validators and
> trusted resources for your friends and neighbors, to help them under-
> stand what's now available for them, and how they can stay healthy
> and safe. . . . Get out and spread the word. This is something that I
> think we'll be able to look back on, just like we do on Medicare and
> Social Security, as really, a cornerstone that improves the security of
> millions of Americans.

Both men recognized resistance. Johnson used the setting of the East Room
to discuss it. Obama spoke on the problem during a telephone conference
with advocates. He called for a grassroots effort to calm fears.

Politics shapes health care reform policy. This process is clearly seen
by comparing liberal and conservative explanations for health care costs,
public programs, and health disparities. To keep this simple, let us compare the language in issue briefs produced by the Center for American
Progress with those from the American Enterprise Institute. The Center
for American Progress reflects a mainstream liberal perspective, while the
American Enterprise Institute reflects a mainstream conservative view.
Curbing health costs was a theme heard on both sides. Each cited similar
data describing the growing annual expenditures. Both groups agreed that
excess costs needed to be contained. Liberals based their response on the
belief that *predatory business practices* contribute to the cost problem.
One example of their approach to curbing these practices is a uniform
medical loss ratio for all insurance plans (Section 2718). Medical loss ratio
refers to a requirement that an insurance company spend a uniform percent
of premium dollars paid by the consumer to purchase health care. Prior to
the ACA, there was no uniform medical loss ratio. Insurance companies
were free to use as much or as little of the premiums to pay for actual care.
Altering the percent of premiums allocated to health care is a strategy
used to maintain shareholder profits. Some companies allocated as little
as 50 percent of premium dollars to pay for health care. The remaining
50 percent was pure profit.

Conservatives control costs by promoting competition among businesses. In general, a company manipulates its pricing structure to compete
for customers. An example of a policy to promote lower costs through

competition is Medicare Part D pharmacy insurance plan pricing. Every year during open enrollment season, Medicare beneficiaries can choose a different pharmacy insurance plan. During this period, companies jockey for customers by promoting their low cost. It is up to the consumer—in this case Medicare enrollee—to look at the formulary associated with a particular cost. Prescription insurance was added to the packet of Medicare benefits in 2007. This benefit is managed by private insurance companies who compete for subscribers within specific geographic areas. Price competition is based on a balance of premiums and benefits. These examples serve to illustrate philosophical differences rather than debate the efficacy of a specific liberal or conservative policy. I will leave that analysis to others. A liberal approach to cost containment *limits predation* by business while the conservative approach *promotes competition* among businesses.

The role of public insurance plans was also debated during ACA development. On a fundamental level, liberals argued for comprehensive insurance for all. Some called it *Medicare for all,* while others spoke of a *public plan* rooted in a commitment to collective responsibility and shared governance. Conservatives promoted expansion of the private insurance markets. Some wanted to eliminate Medicare and provide supplements to purchase insurance in the private markets. Conservative policy was based on a deep mistrust of government, a dedication to individual vigilance, and a belief in the power of free markets. Crafting health care policy to balance these divergent perspectives is not easy. Accommodating a need to diminish health disparities added another level of complexity to the process. Advocates for populations experiencing health disparities understood that neither political group held the answer.

Both government and business have contributed to health disparities in the United States. The U.S. Public Health Service Syphilis Study at Tuskegee is a widely discussed example. Briefly, government scientists blocked access of a group of African American World War I veterans to health care for syphilis for more than 40 years. In the 1930s, when the study began, medical researchers promoted the idea that Negroes were not human and, therefore, not harmed by long-term infection with syphilis. The scientists discounted evidence from observational studies of infection that had already been completed among Scandinavian populations. These studies clearly showed serious consequences: syphilis causes heart and nervous system damage if untreated for a period of years. Predatory business practices have a recent history of creating health care inequity. In April 2009, Quest Diagnostics Incorporated (and its subsidiary, Nichols Institute Diagnostics) paid 300 million dollars under the False Claims

Act to resolve allegations that it provided inaccurate and unreliable parathyroid hormone immunoassay test kits. These kits are used by laboratories throughout the country to measure parathyroid hormone levels in
patients. In this case, the kits were sold for patients in the End Stage Renal
Disease Program administered by Medicare. This benefit provides dialy-
sis to patients with kidney failure. In the United States, minority groups,
low-income persons, and women have the highest rates of kidney failure.
These groups do not have the resources to sue businesses for selling de-
fective items. In these situations, government plays a role in protecting
chronic-care patients from predatory business practices through the False
Claims Act.

A third issue was the debate over the very concept of health disparities. Are disparities a result of individual failure to make good choices?
Does our health care system create the problem? Klick and Satel argue
that there is no evidence that physicians contribute to health disparities.
Their view is opposed by a Government Accounting Office (GAO) study
that was authorized by Senator Bill Frist (R-Tennessee). In the report, the
GAO clearly shows that the physician–patient relationships make a major
contribution to health disparities. Conservatives promoted the view that
personal characteristics of the patient create disparity. Senator John Ensign (R-Nevada), who was a member of the U.S. Senate Finance Committee, articulated the following explanation for differences in health and
proposed a policy solution during the debate:

> Health care is a very personal issue for Americans and choice in
> their coverage should play a vital role. . . . Furthermore Americans
> should be incentivized to lead a healthy lifestyle. Weight manage-
> ment, preventive care, and smoking cessation should be reflected in
> lower insurance rates.

For Senator Ensign, all diseases are a result of personal choice. If policy
penalizes the individual for choices that lead to illness, their health habits
will improve. Pairing individual decisions with economic consequences
is a strategy that will lead to lower health care costs. During the same
Finance Committee debate, Senator Charles Schumer (D-New York) articulated the opposing view:

> Without a public option, you're going to have no competition . . . we
> don't trust the private companies left to their own devices.

In Senator Schumer's view, the choices made by an individual were coun-
terbalanced by the strategies businesses use to increase their profits. In his
remarks, the senator does not explicitly discuss health disparities. Rather,
he argues for a governmental role to protect all consumers from these
practices.

Is health insurance reform a civil rights issue? A room full of health care
reform advocates would agree that health care inequity is a civil rights
issue. These same professionals might not be able to name a specific policy
in the ACA designed to decrease inequity. One or two might mention the
new patient data statutes (Section 4302). With the new data requirements,
hospital administrators will be able to look for differences in care among
groups of patients within their institutions. Someone else might mention
the new National Institute on Minority Health and Health Disparities (Section 10334). A survey of the room's inhabitants would yield a common
definition for civil rights. However, specific ACA policies remain mostly
an abstract concept in the minds of these advocates.

Why don't advocates view the financing of Medicaid as a civil rights
issue? Under the ACA, eligibility for Medicaid will expand to include new
groups (Section 2001). Childless adults whose income is 100 percent of
poverty level will be eligible. Many men with chronic psychiatric illnesses
are in this category. Medicaid is an insurance program administered by
each state. Just like the private insurance plans, it purchases health care.
It differs from private plans in its eligibility requirements and its benefit
packages. Children, pregnant women, impoverished elderly, and the disabled are mandatory populations under Medicaid. Their needs must be
covered first. Under Medicaid, children receive mandatory screenings to
identify impediments to normal development. Families with private insurance do not have vision, hearing, and dental coverage, which is available under Medicaid, for their children unless they purchase it separately.
Under the old rules, young, single men were not eligible for Medicaid
in some states. The states are concerned about the impact that expanded
Medicaid eligibility will have on their budgets. Will Medicaid expansion
reduce health care inequity?

To understand a federal law's intent, begin with the president's discussion of it. Comparing Barack Obama's remarks at the ACA signing
ceremony with those from Lyndon B. Johnson at Medicare's signing
suggests that there is a civil rights potential for the ACA. In addition
to providing clues about the legislative intent, the location and staging
of the signing of a bill reveals very different presidential views about

rewards. In President Obama's view, the content of the ACA is the direct result of his shared experience with millions of Americans. He rewards the faithful:

> Health insurance reform becomes law in the United States. . . . I am signing this reform bill on behalf of my mother, who argued with insurance companies even as she battled cancer in her final days.
> (March 2010, East Room of the White House)

He goes on to name the everyday citizens present at the signing. These citizens include Ryan Smith, a small business owner; Natoma Canfield, a cancer patient dying without health insurance coverage; and Marcelas Owens, an 11-year-old boy whose story of the death of his mother is remarkably similar to Obama's. The signing ceremony—one of several appointments on the presidential schedule that day—was a raucous celebration with applause and shout-outs. The citizen witnesses have a shared experience battling health insurance companies. With the new law, they won a monumental victory. During the signing ceremony, Obama declared that health reform is law:

> [W]hen I sign this bill, all of the overheated rhetoric over reform will finally confront the reality of reform. . . . We are not a nation that scales back its aspirations. We are not a nation that falls prey to doubt or mistrust. We are a nation that faces its challenges and accepts its responsibilities . . . we shape our own destiny.

The atmosphere of the ACA signing starkly contrasts with Johnson's Medicare signing ceremony. Today, time is a limited resource, and even an occasion as momentous as the ACA signing receives no more time than any other afternoon, workday reception in the White House. Johnson, however, devoted 36 hours to activities before and after Medicare signing. His Medicare signing ceremony was a solemn occasion held at the Truman Library in Independence, Missouri. Johnson used the occasion to continue the process of recruiting support for the new law. By signing the legislation in Missouri, he shared the historical spotlight with opponents in a very conservative area of the United States. Rather than mentioning the stories of individual citizens who will benefit from the legislation, he spoke of President Truman and 23 other federal officials—senators, representatives, and cabinet members. By including the elected officials in the historic occasion, he created photo opportunities.

He also used a moral appeal to shame community leaders into support for the Medicaid portion of the law. In President Johnson's view, health care is a moral obligation. It continues the legacy begun by President Truman:

> maintain and improve the health of all Americans . . . this is not just our tradition—or the tradition of the Democratic Party—or even the tradition of the nation. It is as old as the day it was first commanded: "Thou shalt open thine hand wide unto thy brother, thy poor, to thy needy, in thy land."

What else distinguishes Obama's and Johnson's views on health care inequity? For Johnson, respect for elders was a primary motivation for Medicare:

> These people are our prideful responsibility and they are entitled . . . to the best medical protection available. Not one of these citizens should ever be abandoned to the indignity of charity.

For Obama, basic health care security is the main aim of the new law:

> as soon as I sign this bill . . . the core principle that everybody should have some basic security when it comes to their health care [is enshrined].

How does each president respond to the idea that health care reform is controversial? All students of government know that making new laws is just a first step. To realize the promise of the law, citizens must use it. Does either president address this need for citizens to put aside their concerns and embrace the new law? Did either president use a civil rights rationale to persuade reluctant adopters? We know that the American Medical Association was a vocal opponent of the Medicare bill. In his signing remarks, Johnson described a meeting with the American Medical Association leadership:

> yesterday, at the request of some of my friends, I met with the leaders of the American Medical Association to seek their assistance in advancing the cause of one of the greatest professions of all—the medical profession—in helping us to maintain and to improve the health of all Americans.

Johnson did not describe the content of that closed-door discussion. It was rumored that he promised financial incentives to gain support. This is a contrast to Obama's approach to the American Medical Association. On June 21, 2009, President Obama traveled to Chicago to address the American Medical Association in a public forum. His remarks carry a specific message of cost containment to the group:

> the cost of our health care is a threat to our economy . . . an escalating burden on our families and businesses. It is a ticking time bomb for the federal budget . . . it's unsustainable for the United States. Reform is not a luxury, but a necessity . . . the cost of not acting is greater . . . health care reform is the single most important thing we can do for America's long-term fiscal health . . . part of the reason [prior efforts have failed] has been the fierce opposition fueled by some interest groups and lobbyists—opposition that has used fear tactics to paint any effort as an attempt to socialize medicine.
>
> . . . we can build a health care system that allows you to be physicians instead of administrators and accountants . . . we need to upgrade our medical records by switching from a paper to an electronic system of record keeping . . . this means less paper pushing and lower administrative costs . . . a system of incentives where more tests and services are provided the more we pay . . . it is a model that rewards quantity of care rather than quality . . . gives you every incentive to order that extra Magnetic Resonance Image or Electrocardiogram.
>
> . . . You did not enter this profession to be bean counters and paper pushers . . . reform the way we compensate doctors and hospitals. We need to bundle payments so you aren't paid for every single treatment you offer . . . but instead are paid for how you treat the overall disease . . . create incentives for physicians to team up . . . it results in a healthier patient.
>
> . . . rethink the cost of a medical education . . . we need to improve the quality of medical information making its way to doctors and patients.
>
> . . . even when we do know what works, we are often not making the most of it. [In] Cincinnati Children's Hospital . . . the quality of care for cystic fibrosis patients shot up after the hospital began to incorporate suggestions from patients. . . . My signature on a bill is not enough. I need your help, doctors. . . . I will listen to you and work with you to pursue reform that works for you.

The current state of inequality in health care begs the question: Can health insurance reform serve a civil rights agenda? The health care inequity framework is larger than a black-and-white view. It includes low-wage workers, persons with limited English proficiency, and women to name a few groups. The ACA is first and foremost an overhaul of the health insurance business model. Do current health insurance business practices make a measurable contribution to patterns of care inequity among a broader group of Americans? Will reframing business practices diminish inequities among groups of insured workers, young adults, and entrepreneurs? Is medical fraud a contributor to inequity in the United States? With this expanded frame, can we see a link between business practices and inequities in the U.S. health care markets? The ACA's text does not directly link health insurance business practices with health care inequities. The connection between historical insurance business practices and present-day inequity is a question worthy of its own book-length analysis. This book will emphasize the ACA's potential to address today's issues.

The *political will* to pass the ACA was based on a health care narrative involving limited access, excessive cost, and consumer dissatisfaction. With the exception of Johnson's success in 1964, presidents dating back to Truman lacked an essential, personal ingredient. What was the campaign message that built support for the ACA? During the presidential campaign in fall of 2008, the following health care narrative emerged:

> health care—this isn't about politics for me. This is personal. I'm thinking today about my mother. She died of ovarian cancer at the age of fifty three. She fought valiantly, and endured the pain and chemotherapy with grace and good humor. But I'll never forget how she spent the final months of her life. At a time when she should have been focused on getting well, at a time when she should have been taking stock of her life and taking comfort in her family, she was lying in a hospital bed, fighting with her insurance company because they didn't want to cover her treatment. They claimed that her cancer was a pre-existing condition. . . . So I know something about the heartbreak caused by our health care system.
>
> (Obama, Newport News, Virginia, October 4, 2008)

Some voters lived this story. Others knew someone engaged in the struggle. Similar stories were shared in rallies, on blogs, and in speeches. Obama's experience with his mom's death from ovarian cancer defines his approach to health care policy. She had insurance but was denied access to life-sustaining care. The story links life-threatening illness, soul-sucking paperwork, and administrative obstinacy.

In a different way, Johnson drew on his personal experience with educational systems and federal laws to guide his policy approach to health reform. Johnson had personal experience with family financial failure. He was grounded in civil rights as a teacher of Mexican American children and had a deep understanding of southern segregation. The Medicare and Medicaid Act of 1965 reflected an appreciation of state government he learned as the state director of the National Youth Administration in Texas. He was, first and foremost, a *son of the South*. His vision of civil rights and the Great Society created the social safety net that millions rely on today. In the first few lines of Medicare, health care is defined as an entitlement.

In a 2007 speech, then Senator Obama foreshadowed the ACA reforms designed to address health care inequity:

[W]e can't afford another disappointing charade in 2008. It's not only tiresome, it's wrong. [It is] wrong when businesses have to lay off one employee because they can't afford the health care of another. Wrong when a parent cannot take a sick child to the doctor because they cannot afford the bill that comes with it. Wrong when forty six million Americans have no health care at all. In a country that spends more on health care than any other nation on Earth, it's just wrong.

And yet, in recent years, what's caught the attention of those who haven't always been in favor of reform is the realization that this crisis . . . [is] economically untenable. . . . You know the statistics. Family premiums are up by nearly eighty seven percent over the last five years, growing five times faster than workers' wages. Deductibles are up fifty percent. Co-payments for care and prescriptions are through the roof.

Nearly eleven million Americans who are already insured spent more than a quarter of their salary on health care last year. And over half of all family bankruptcies today are caused by medical bills. Almost half of all small businesses no longer offer health care to their workers . . . others . . . lay off workers or shut their doors for good. Some of the biggest corporations in America, giants of industry like

General Motors and Ford, are watching foreign competitors based in countries with universal health care run circles around them, with a General Motors car containing twice as much health care cost as a Japanese car.

They tell us it's too expensive to cover the uninsured, but they don't mention that every time an American without health insurance walks into an emergency room, we pay even more. Our family's premiums are nine hundred and twenty two dollars higher because of the cost of care for the uninsured.

We pay fifteen billion dollars more in taxes because of the cost of care for the uninsured. And it's trapped us in a vicious cycle. As the uninsured cause premiums to rise, more employers drop coverage. As more employers drop coverage, more people become uninsured, and premiums rise even further . . .

[W]hen you see what the health care crisis is doing to our families, to our economy, to our country, you realize that caution is what's costly. Inaction is what's risky. Doing nothing is what's impossible when it comes to health care in America.

At a time when businesses are facing increased competition and workers rarely stay with one company throughout their lives, we also have to ask if the employer based system of health care, itself is still the best for providing insurance to all Americans. We have to ask what we can do to provide more Americans with preventative [sic] care, which would mean fewer doctor's visits and less cost down the road. We should make sure that every single child who's eligible is signed up for the children's health insurance program, and the federal government should make sure that our states have the money to make that happen.

Each segment of the ACA is outlined in this speech. Market reforms, employer concerns, and the responsibilities shared by individuals and society are placed within the context of health care inequity. The candidate, however, does not articulate a connection between race and health care inequity. Where does the historical legacy of discrimination fit into health care reform? Does Obama acknowledge a role for racism? In a speech entitled "A More Perfect Union," then candidate Obama described his perspective on race, its place in current American society, and its priority within health reform:

race is an issue that . . . this nation cannot afford to ignore right now. We would be making [a] mistake . . .—to simplify and stereotype and amplify the negative to the point that it distorts reality. The fact is that the comments that . . . the complexities of race in this country . . . [Are] a part of our union that we have yet to perfect? . . . [I]f we simply retreat into our respective corners; we will never be able to come together and solve challenges like health care.

> (Obama on Race, March 18, 2008,
> in Philadelphia, Pennsylvania)

In Obama's experience, reform consists of changing insurance practices. Ban the rules that deny care or delay treatment. Give health care purchasers what they pay for—care when needed. Each provision confronts the gotcha narrative. What is a gotcha? You are involved in a gotcha narrative when you make any of the following statements. Why cannot I have the medicine my doctor ordered? *Gotcha!* Why is not my pregnancy covered? *Gotcha!* My seven-year-old son, Billy, needs this surgery to correct a problem we have been treating since birth. What do you mean the lifetime limit for treatment has been reached? *Gotcha!* The fine print in your insurance policy limits care when you are at your most vulnerable.

ACA policy is not a *health care for all* model. It uses the language of insurance markets. Market excess is curbed by regulations. Market regulation, not civil rights or social safety nets, defines ACA policy. These are all items that health insurance consumers want in a policy. At the very beginning in Title I, Subtitle A the law specifies:

- No limits on medical payouts in a calendar year and policy lifetime (Section 2711)
- No capricious cancellation of health care coverage (Section 2712)
- Required coverage for preventive services (Section 2713)
- Required coverage for dependent kids within families (Section 2714)
- No deceptive communication in marketing insurance plans (Section 2715)
- No discrimination based on salary among employer-sponsored plans (Section 2716)
- Oversight to ensure safety and quality in health care (Section 2717)
- No excess profiteering (Section 2718)
- Standardized appeal process (Section 2719)

If civil rights legislation made discrimination illegal, is there any reason to think that the current pattern of health care inequity is race based? This fundamental question will be explored in each chapter.

## BIBLIOGRAPHY

Beardsley, Edward H. *A History of Neglect: Health Care for Blacks and Mill Workers in the Twentieth-Century South*. Knoxville: The University of Tennessee Press, 1987.

Bennett, Paul G. "VA Health Economics Bulletin: Guidebook for Research Use of Paid Data," edited by Health Economics Resource Center, 2. Menlo Park, 2009.

Blanchard, Janice, and Nicole Lurie. "R-E-S-P-E-C-T: Patient Reports of Disrespect in the Health Care Setting and Its Impact on Care." *Journal of Family Practice* 53, no. 9 (2004): 721. Published electronically September 2004, http://www.jfponline.com/pdf%2F5309%2F5309JFP_OriginalResearch.pdf.

Center for Medicare and Medicaid Services. "Premier Hospital Historical Data," https://www.cms.gov/HospitalQualitynits/40_HospitalPremierHistoricalData.asp.

Claxton, Gary, Bianca DiJulio, Benjamin Finder, Janet Lundy, Megan McHugh, Awo Osei-Anto, Heidi Whitmore, Jeremy Pickreign, and Jon Gabel. "Employer Health Benefits: 2009 Summary of Findings." Kaiser Family Foundation, Health Research & Education Trust, National Opinion Research Center, 2009.

Cline, Jane, Kevin McCarty, Roger Sevigny, Susan Voss, Kim Holland, Sandy Praeger. "Letter to Commissioner Alfred W. Gross of America's Health Insurance Plans; Re: Key Remaining Concerns Regarding MLR, MLR Health Care Quality Initiatives, and a Transition Plan to Address Potential Market Disruption." National Association of Insurance Commissions & Center for Insurance Research and Policy, July 6, 2010.

Cooper-Patrick, Lisa, Joseph J. Gallo, Junius J. Gonzalez, Hong Thi Vu, Neil R. Powe, Christine Nelson, and Daniel E. Ford. "Race, Gender, and Partnership in the Patient–Physician Relationship." *Journal of the American Medical Association* 282, no. 6 (1999): 583–89. Published electronically 1999. doi:10.1001/jama.282.6.583. http://jama.ama-assn.org/content/282/6/583.abstract.

Deloitte Center for Health Solutions. "2009 Survey of Health Care Consumers: Key Findings, Strategic Implications." Deloitte LLP, http://www.deloitte.com/us/2009consumersurvey.

Department of Veterans Affairs. "Veteran Population Model (Vetpop 2007)." Office of the Assistant Secretary for Policy and Planning, Office of Policy, 2008.

Dominitz, Jason A., Charles Maynard, Kevin G. Billingsley, and Edward J. Boyko. "Race, Treatment, and Survival of Veterans with Cancer of the Distal Esophagus and Gastric Cardia." *Medical Care* 40, no. 1, Supplement: Racial-Disparities Research in Veterans Healthcare Administration (2002): I14–I26.

Ghazal, Maria. "Rin 0938-Aq17 Comments Re: Proposed Rule for Medicare Program; Availability of Medicare Data for Performance Measurement, 76 Fed. Reg. 33566 (June 8, 2011)," edited by *Business Roundtable,* 5, 2011.

Hynes, Denise M., Duane Cowper, Michael Kerr, Joseph Kubal, and Patricia A. Murphy. "Database and Informatics Support Queri: Current Systems and Future Needs." *Medical Care* 38, no. QUERI Supplement (2000): I114–I128.

Iglehart, John K. "Medicare, Graduate Medical Education, and New Policy Directions." *New England Journal of Medicine* 359, no. 6 (2008): 8.

Johnson, Lyndon Baines. "President Lyndon B. Johnson's Radio and Television Remarks Upon Signing the Civil Rights Bill July 2, 1964." *Public Papers of the Presidents of the United States: Lyndon B. Johnson, 1963–64.* Volume II, entry 446. Washington, DC: Government Printing Office, 1965.

Johnson, Lyndon Baines. "President Lyndon B. Johnson's Remarks with President Truman at the Signing in Independence of the Medicare Bill." *Public Papers of the Presidents of the United States: Lyndon B. Johnson, 1965.* Volume II, entry 394. Washington, DC: Government Printing Office, 1965.

Johnson, Randel K., and Katie Mahoney. "Re: Proposed Rule Regarding the Availability of Medicare Data for Performance Measurement," edited by U.S. Chamber of Commerce. U.S. Chamber Website, 2011.

Jones, James H. *Bad Blood: The Tuskegee Syphilis Experiment.* New York: The Free Press, 1993.

Kressin, Nancy R., Ulrike Boehmer, Dan Berlowitz, Cindy L. Christiansen, Arkadiy Pitman, and Judith A. Jones. "Racial Variations in Dental Procedures: The Case of Root Canal Therapy Versus Tooth Extraction." *Medical Care* 41, no. 11 (2003): 1256–61.

Levinson, Daniel R. "Adverse Events in Hospitals: National Incidence among Medicare Beneficiaries." OEI-06-09-00090. Office of the Inspector General. Washington, DC, November 2010.

Ly, Dan P., Lenny Lopez, Thomas Isaac, and Ashisha K. Jha. "How Do Black-Serving Hospitals Perform on Patient Safety Indicators? Implications for National Public Reporting and Pay-for-Performance." *Medical Care* 48, no. 12 (2010): 1133–37. Published electronically December 2010. doi:10.1097/MLR.0b013e3181f81c7e.

Miles, Toni P., and David McBride. "World War I Origins of the Syphilis Epidemic among 20th Century Black Americans: A Biohistorical Analysis." *Social Science Medicine* 45, no. 1 (1997): 61–69.

Milligan, Chuck. "Reshaping Medicaid." Discussion draft for Health Summit. National Governors Association, 2009, http://www.nga.org/files/live/sites/ NGA/files/pdf/1003HEALTHSUMMITRESHAPINGMEDICAID. PDF.

Obama, Barack H. "A More Perfect Union." *Huffington Post,* http://www.huffing tonpost.com/2008/03/18/obama-race-speech-read-th_n_92077.html.

Obama, Barack H. "Obama Holds Teleconference on Affordable Care Act." *Washington Post,* http://projects.washingtonpost.com/obama-speeches/speech/ 411/.

Obama, Barack H. *Obama Signs Health-Care Bill into Law.* In Obama's words, edited by Jackie Kazil Wilson Andrews, Nathaniel Vaughn Kelso, Sarah Lovenheim, Ryan O'Neil, Paul Volpe, and Karen Yourish. Washington, DC: *The Washington Post,* 2010.

Oliver, Adam. "The Veterans Health Administration: An American Success Story?" *Milbank Quarterly* 85, no. 1 (2007): 5–35. Published electronically January.

Petersen, Laura A., Steven M. Wright, Eric D. Peterson, and Jennifer Daley. "Impact of Race on Cardiac Care and Outcomes in Veterans with Acute Myocardial Infarction." *Medical Care* 40, no. 1, Supplement Racial Disparities Research in the Veterans Health Care Administration (2002): 186–196.

Robertson, Russel G. (Chair). "Advancing Primary Care." Council on Graduate Medical Education. Twentieth Report, December 2010, http://www.aafp. org/online/etc/medialib/aafp_org/documents/press/2011-match-media-kit/ cogme-advancing-primary-care.Par.0001.File.tmp/COGME-20threport-2011-Exec-Summ.pdf.

Russell, Lesley. "How Health Care Reform Benefits People of Color." Center for American Progress, http://www.americanprogress.org/issues/2011/01/ war_minorities.html.

Satcher, David, George E. Fryer, Jessica McCann, Adewale Troutman, Steven H. Woolf, and George Rust. "What If We Were Equal? A Comparison of the Black–White Mortality Gap in 1960 and 2000." *Health Affairs* 24, no. 2 (2000): 459–64.

Satel, Sally, and Jonathan Klick. *The Health Disparities Myth: Diagnosing the Treatment Gap.* Washington, DC: American Enterprise Institute Press, 2006.

Towers Watson. "Express Scripts' Merger with Medco Health Solutions: Potential Implications for Employers," 2011.

U.S. Bureau of Labor Statistics. "On Benefits by Wage Level: Survey Finds That Employer Provided Benefits Vary with Earnings." Program Perspectives, U.S. Department of Labor, 2010.

U.S. Congress, 79th. "Hospital Survey and Construction Act (Hill Burton Act)," 79, PL79-725.

Vaughn, Thomas E., Kimberly D. McCoy, Bonnie J. BootsMiller, Robert F. Woolson, Bernard Sorofman, Toni Tripp-Reimer, Jonathan Perlin, and Bradley

N. Doebbeling. "Organizational Predictors of Adherence to Ambulatory Care Screening Guidelines." *Medical Care* 40, no. 40 (2002): 1172–85.

Wailoo, Keith. *Dying in the City of the Blues: Sickle Cell Anemia and the Politics of Race and Health.* Chapel Hill, NC: The University of North Carolina Press, 2001.

Yi, Song G. "Consumer-Driven Health Care: What Is It and What Does It Mean for Employees and Employers?," Bureau of Labor Statistics, 2010.

# CHAPTER 2

## Beyond Medicaid

Medicaid is a public insurance plan. It operates at the intersection of race, social class, economics, and local politics. There are no national conversations about Medicaid. There are 50 separate shouting matches. Each debate reflects regional differences in population, taxing authority, and the perception of individual responsibility. In one bundle, Medicaid is expected to provide the entire spectrum of health care needs—acute care, hospital care, long-term services, early-screening prevention and detection in childhood, and medical supplies. There is no comparable business model of cradle-to-grave coverage in the private insurance markets. If you are an impoverished pregnant woman without health insurance, Medicaid can pay your maternity care bills. If you are a child living in a household without insurance, Medicaid is designed to cover your health care. If you are blind, disabled, or an impoverished elder, Medicaid is obligated to support services that bolster independence. Implementation of the ACA and its Medicaid provisions between now and 2019 will shape the future of health care inequities.

### CONSUMER VOICES AND MEDICAID

In a consumer society, satisfaction with goods and services is the pathway to increased sales and, ultimately, increased profits. For the first time in U.S. history, Section 3001 of the ACA links payment to consumer satisfaction with health care. The Hospital Value Based Purchasing Program provides incentive payments to hospitals meeting performance standards.

Hospital performance on the Consumer Assessment of Healthcare Providers and Systems (CAHPS) survey is one type of measurement that will drive payment. The voices of patients, particularly those on Medicaid, are usually discounted in any discussion of policy. Representative Barney Frank (D-Massachusetts) has commented on the exclusion of poor people from a conversation that is vital to their lives:

> For many of those who had historically supported welfare programs in the broadest sense, it was perfectly reasonable to enact legislation in which poor people were the objects of efforts to assist them. But when others suggested that the poor should not simply be the objects of these programs but also the subjects—that they should be actively involved in shaping the programs, making decisions about how to spend the money, etc.—some of the previous supporters reconsidered.

If asked, what would persons covered by Medicaid say about the program? A clear policy emphasis running throughout the ACA is payment reform. Consumer satisfaction is a part of the payment-reform process. The goal is to improve the *quality* of health care. Congressman Frank's comment suggests that even advocates are not comfortable with actively involving the ideas of *actual Medicaid recipients*. What would *Medicaid clients* say about the quality of care they receive? Is this different from the experience and opinions of persons with private health insurance? Do we have a way of knowing the answers to these questions? The short answer to the last question is "Yes." Funded and administered by the U.S. Agency for Healthcare Research and Quality, the CAHPS is a family of standardized surveys designed to capture consumer experiences with the performance of health insurance plans in both the public and private markets. These surveys are designed to support the *consumer's* information needs. They are the product of more than 10 years of scientific testing and designed to provide information to the public. This means that anyone can use the survey data free of charge. For more details on the development of CAHPS, the reader should visit the website of the Agency for Healthcare Research and Quality: www.ahrq.gov.

ACA payment-reform policy uses measures of consumer satisfaction to reward health care quality. Whether your business is a five-star hotel or a fast-food hamburger franchise, consumer satisfaction is critical. Do any groups of consumers believe that they receive high-quality health care? The National Committee for Quality Assurance uses CAHPS data from members of public and private insurance plans in its ranking system. One item—*overall rating of health plan*—illustrates the perspective that CAHPS brings to the discussion of Medicaid. With this question, members rate their health plan on a scale of 0 to 10. A rating of zero implies the worst health plan possible, and a rating of 10 implies the best. The National Committee for Quality Assurance provides yearly reports comparing plans on this and other CAHPS measures. There is clear evidence of consumer dissatisfaction with Medicaid in the 2010 report. Among Medicaid members, 33 percent rate their plan as a seven or less. For private plans, 25 percent of members rate their health plan as a seven or less. Medicare members have the lowest levels of dissatisfaction (15%). While we do not know the true cause of dissatisfaction, we can speculate that government management does not explain differences between Medicaid and private plans. In most states, Medicaid is a public plan that is *privately managed*. In contrast, Medicare is a *public plan* with *government management*. Oklahoma, Arizona, Alabama, and Mississippi are the only states where the state government manages Medicaid. The remaining states process Medicaid claims through a patchwork of contracts with managed-care businesses. In essence, when consumers rate their health plan, they are usually rating the performance of a private business.

The CAHPS survey has an item measuring *ease of obtaining customer service*. Ease is linked to health care access. Lack of access to care is a prime contributor to health care inequity. The ease rating of consumers range from *always* to *never*. Nationwide, 20 percent of Medicaid health plan members report that it is *never* easy to obtain service. Again, Medicare beneficiaries are the least likely group to report that it is never easy (14%). Sixteen percent of private plan members report that it is never easy to obtain service. If we looked at a single state and compared member ratings of private and Medicaid plans, would we see a different picture of customer service? New York commercial plans statewide and the Healthfirst Medicaid managed plan have similar levels of dissatisfaction. Twenty percent of Healthfirst members report that health care is *sometimes* or *never* easy to obtain. What would New York state health plan members tell Governor Andrew Cuomo and Healthfirst President and CEO Pat Wang? They would say that the overall quality of service in New York health plans—not just Medicaid—needs work. Although 20 percent seems like a small number, it is important to understand that customer service is a surrogate for access to office visits. When office visits are difficult to obtain, the alternative is an emergency room visit. In 2007, almost five million persons were enrolled in Medicaid in New York. If 20 percent of plan members have difficulty obtaining customer service, then almost one million people might be inclined to access the emergency room for routine care.

The larger society also voices its values through the structure of Medicaid. How does Medicaid reflect the high value we place on individual responsibility? All adults in the United States are expected to attain economic independence sometime between the ages of 18 and 25 years. Throughout a work life of 40 to 50 years, we are encouraged to amass sufficient resources to meet day-to-day needs and anticipate our dependency in old age. These prototypical adults are expected to procure resources for themselves as well as any dependents they choose to shelter. This model of adulthood is based on an assumption of ability and good fortune. These abilities are grounded in a quality education and rewarded with monetary value in the marketplace. In planning for the future, people also often assume good fortune. This scenario does not accommodate events that derail education or devalue one's labor. Employer-sponsored health insurance is one measure of past or potential market value. Adults without jobs generally do not have health insurance—unless they are married to workers with employer-sponsored insurance. Low-wage workers are also less likely to have health insurance. These adults may have children. They also come in a variety of ages. Some are young adults attempting to leave their parental homes. Others are at the end of their work lives. Some of these adults cannot perform in a workplace that increasingly emphasizes cognitive skills over physical abilities. All of these adults and their dependents are potential candidates for Medicaid. Medicaid is a health insurance program that values children, pregnant women, the disabled, the blind, and the elderly. Eligibility for Medicaid begins where our market value–based system of health insurance ends. These markets reflect future and past contributions to the economy.

Does the structure of Medicaid create winners and losers in health care access? After all, medical need is not a criterion for eligibility for most Medicaid plans. Medicaid is one of those government programs that confuse people. Many hear *Medicaid* but think *Medicare*. *Medicaid* equals *State Health Care Aid*. Access to Medicaid is defined differently in each state. Its benefit package varies from state to state. States receive a calculated funding match from the federal government to administer the local Medicaid program. *Whom does Medicaid serve?* The answer to this question becomes simpler when the program is placed in the larger history of social welfare. One of the first programs in this history was the Statute of Laborers in England (1348). It made a distinction between the *worthy poor* (the aged, handicapped, widows, and dependent children) and the *unworthy poor* (able-bodied but unemployed adults). Current criteria for Medicaid eligibility include mandatory populations—children, pregnant women, people with disabilities, the aged, and the blind. States can decide whether to serve childless adults as *optional* populations. Although Medicaid is defined as a public insurance plan, most states administer their programs through a series of joint public–private contracts. States pay a managed-care organization to negotiate for health care with providers. There is also historical precedence for this model. European workhouses in the 1600s provided care to very young children, the handicapped, and very old people through contracts with entrepreneurs. Can a public program managed by commercial interests be reformed to improve the current picture of health care inequity?

Before we can answer any questions, we must be able to identify Medicaid in an individual state. This is not so simple. A similar problem was described by Arthur C. Clarke in his story entitled *The Nine Billion Names of God*. Monks in a Tibetan lamasery sought to list all the names of God. It takes them almost three centuries to complete the list. Once they get them all, the universe begins to disappear. Medicaid plans across the United States present a similar nomenclature challenge. Think for a second: What is Medicaid called in your area? If we get all the names together, will Medicaid as we know it cease to exist? These plans have a number of names *within* each state because Medicaid is really a family of plans. In Oklahoma, some of the names for Medicaid are *SoonerCare Choice, SoonerCare Health Management Program,* and *Child Health*. SoonerCare Choice provides primary care in a *medical home*. SoonerCare Health Management Program is a chronic disease management plan. Child Health is an early and periodic screening, diagnosis, and treatment plan for children aged 20 years and younger. These names are unique to Oklahoma. If you go north to Kansas or south to Texas, you will encounter names like *MediKan* and *HealthWave* in Kansas; *State of Texas Access Reform* (STAR) and the *Children's Health Insurance Program* (CHIP) in Texas. The vast number of names of Medicaid makes any discussion of health care inequity and Medicaid difficult. Why so many names? This nomenclature does not reflect consumer choices. It reflects the different plans and financing within the larger state Medicaid program.

To move beyond a conversation limited to Medicaid and discuss health care inequity, we must identify persons on both sides of the eligibility criteria. Why? The answer to the health care inequity question is different for persons eligible for Medicaid and those who are not. Eligibility draws a line—inequity of access. Medical need exists on either side of the

eligibility line, but access to health care may or may not. Medicaid eligibility has the hallmarks of English law: the worthy poor. Medically needy
but ineligible persons are branded as able-bodied. Medically needy but
Medicaid ineligible persons experience health care inequity. What about
the eligible individuals? Does Medicaid diminish health care inequity for
eligible persons? The short answer is—*Yes*. Medicaid *does* improve access to health care—particularly for kids. During the period 2002 to 2006,
rural kids enrolled in SoonerCare saw a 35 percent decrease in hospitalization for asthma. This trend among rural kids in Oklahoma indicates an
access to emerging treatments. If Medicaid access improves health care
access, why are there criteria to determine eligibility? To control costs. In
fact, Medicaid policy employs many of the same strategies used by private
insurance plans—limiting benefits and controlling enrollment in the plan.
Unlike private plans, states do not have the luxury of increasing the dollars that beneficiaries can contribute out of pocket. Formerly, states have
managed this fiscal barrier by ratcheting the allowable income for eligibility up or down. In lean fiscal years, one had to be *poorer*. In better times,
states could increase the income eligibility and allow more workers into
the program. Low-wage workers clearly experience health care inequity
due to fluctuating Medicaid eligibility. The issue is not severity of medical
need. The issue is income-based eligibility.

Fluctuating Medicaid eligibility creates health care inequity. Since 1996,
there has been a policy battle between groups trying to expand eligibility
for Medicaid and those trying to control Medicaid's impact on state budgets. The stakes are high for this policy battle. In the United States, almost
40 percent of births are supported with Medicaid. Without this support
for prenatal and maternal care, our infant mortality rate would be higher
than it is. The tension between priorities is reflected in the maximum income level allowed for access to Medicaid by pregnant women. For example, Oklahoma in 1996 had three separate income maximums. Pregnant
women were eligible for coverage at 150 percent of the federal poverty
level (FPL). This was slightly higher than the required federal minimum
in 1996 of 133 percent of the FPL. In Oklahoma, children aged one to six
years were eligible for Medicaid if the household income was 133 percent
of the FPL. This was same as the federal minimum for children in this age
range in 1996. Oklahoma's eligibility standard for children aged six years
and older was 100 percent of the FPL—the same as the federal minimum.
The Balanced Budget Act of 1997 expanded Medicaid eligibility for children up to age 15 in households with an income at 185 percent of the FPL.
By 2002, all children up to age 19 were eligible. In 2006, Oklahoma used

the 100 percent of FPL standard to set eligibility for pregnant women and kids. Forty-two other states had higher levels. Many set the bar at 300 percent of FPL. Did expanding household eligibility improve health for children in the Medicaid program of the other 42 states? According to the Mathematica Policy Research survey group (Mathematica), most trends in the rates of preventable hospitalization among children aged 0 to 19 were not statistically significant during the period 2003 to 2006. The exceptions include a significant decline in asthma-related hospitalizations among male rural enrollees. Did fluctuating eligibility contribute to preventable hospitalizations? Will the ACA make a measurable impact on preventable hospitalizations? The ACA increases Medicaid's reach to a larger pool of low-income households through a *Medicaid expansion* (Title II, Subsection c). The expansion makes income eligibility categories broader.

What about medical need outside of Medicaid eligibility? Workers whose jobs do not offer insurance include small businesses with fewer than 15 employees; service industry workers like waitresses, maids, and cooks; and individual entrepreneurs. Anyone who is self-employed has the same dilemma. Although these workers could purchase individual insurance plans, they usually cannot afford the premiums. With these plans, there are two strategies open to consumers to keep the cost of premiums low. One strategy is to limit benefits. The other is to set a high monetary threshold before the benefits start. These choices are a personal reality for adults living between employer-sponsored and state-supported health insurance. The choices become increasingly problematic for workers with children. The 2007 Behavioral Risk Factor Surveillance System provides data showing that low-wage workers in states like Oklahoma are more likely to delay their health care needs if they have children. Forty-seven percent of low-wage workers with children report foregoing a doctor visit because of cost. These reports from parents in low-wage jobs are independent of race. Black and white parents are equally likely to forego screening mammograms, diabetes, blood lipid tests, or diabetes tests. Reports of delayed medical care are likely for parents of all educational levels—those with no high school as well as those with college education. Prior to ACA Medicaid expansion, enrollment was not an option for newly unemployed workers. The choice to delay care was most common for newly unemployed workers. The recession of 2008 caused the most layoffs for middle-aged workers. Many of these parents have children in middle and high school. Parents delay care at the point in chronic disease diagnosis when it is most successfully controlled with conservative measures. The consequences of delay for these parents are a higher risk of dying. This risk persists over a prolonged period. Most deaths among workers between the ages of 45 and 64 occur after individuals have gained either public or private health insurance. If allowed to happen, the expansion of Medicaid in 2014 will improve access for this group of U.S. adults.

In fact, access to any plan in Medicaid is based on family income and applicant characteristics. The current strategy to broaden access to the limited pool of Medicaid dollars is accomplished by creating a number of *single-benefit plans* (SBPs). The idea is to provide some services with limited cost in each state. Eligibility for these plans is determined by a separate process for each plan. Applicants commonly find that they are eligible for some SBPs within Medicaid but not others. For example, many states have a plan that only provides contraception. There are 36 states with this type of plan. Not all states offer the same contraceptive benefits. Medicaid coverage of sexually transmitted disease *testing* is only available in 11 states. Medicaid-supported *treatment* for the sexually transmitted disease is only available in nine states. Yes, two states will *test* for but not *treat* a sexually transmitted disease. The contraceptive-only plan, one of the SBPs, does not cover other medical needs; for example, if you are an enrollee in the contraceptive-only plan and have diabetes, you get birth control but not diabetes treatment; if you are injured in an accident, you get contraception but not payment for the treatment that your injuries require. There are SBPs for cancer screening (covering breast and cervical cancer only), chronic renal disease, prescription assistance, and medical transportation. Applicants can be eligible for these single benefits but not for comprehensive medical care. This problem is most acute for men between the ages of 18 and 64. In some states, men are eligible for the Medicaid contraception SBP—essentially sterilization—but nothing else. Men with schizophrenia or bipolar disorder as young adults are usually not eligible for any state Medicaid plans until their illness has become chronic and unstable. Unemployed, childless, middle-aged workers who can no longer afford to pay Consolidated Omnibus Budget Reconciliation Act (COBRA) premiums are not eligible for primary care through Medicaid in most states. The ACA has defined a minimum packet of benefits (Title I—Essential Benefits) and essentially eliminated SBPs for private insurance plans. Should Medicaid move away from SBPs? SBPs are a mixed blessing. They create both inequity and access. If an SBP is a bad idea in the private markets, is it not a bad idea in public plans? Although Obama's speeches on health care reform never reference Medicaid, Title II in the ACA was dedicated solely to reforming this public program. The law is silent, however, about SBP in Medicaid.

How does Medicaid policy connect to a market-based view of health care inequity? The answer to this question has implications for both state governors and Medicaid beneficiaries. During the period 1995 to 2005, the U.S. national average for Medicaid expenditures as a proportion of total state expenses rose from almost 10 percent to more than 13 percent. If asked, each group might define inequity and cost in different terms. In media and policy circles, the conversation surrounding Medicaid only involves government officials and the institutions delivering Medicaid-supported health care. The opinion of the consumer is not solicited. To illustrate the divide between thinking about state budgets and serving beneficiaries, consider the New York State Medicaid Redesign Team. In January 2011, the newly elected governor, Andrew M. Cuomo, announced the formation of a *Medicaid Redesign Team*. This group was tasked to find ways to save money within Medicaid for the state budget for the fiscal year 2011–2012. The team includes up to 25 voting members appointed by the governor. Members are drawn from state officers with relevant expertise, two members of the New York State Assembly, two members of the New York State Senate, leaders with expertise in the health care industry, and business and consumer leaders. In his announcement, Governor Cuomo said:

> New York's bloated Medicaid program, which spends at a rate more than twice the national average, must be reformed to help our state begin to make ends meet. This new team has been tasked with finding ways to save Medicaid money which will finally give taxpayers a needed break.
>
> (January 5, 2011)

Healthfirst CEO Pat Wang acknowledged Governor Cuomo's announcement:

> I am tremendously encouraged by the governor's recognition of the need for a fundamental restructuring of the state's Medicaid program and his commitment to do so in partnership with providers, workers, and consumers. He is right in saying that better coordination [is needed] for the care of people with complex conditions.
>
> (January 5, 2011)

Healthfirst is a Medicaid managed care company. Its primary business is management of public plans for New York, Florida, and other states. Wang's comments represent the perspective of an insurance company. Another group on the Medicaid Redesign Team is *Medicaid Matters New York*. Medicaid Matters New York is a statewide, consumer-oriented coalition that advocates on behalf of New York's Medicaid program and the people it serves. Lara Kassel, the coordinator for this group, was also appointed as a member of the team. Medicaid Matters New York's top five priorities for the team are:

- Maintaining benefits while eliminating barriers to care and services.
- Maintaining eligibility levels and streamlining enrollment processes.
- Ensuring transparency and accountability in all Medicaid spending.
- Avoiding across-the-board cuts to Medicaid providers.
- Giving priority to *safety net providers* over better resourced, less accessible providers. Safety net providers serve Medicaid consumers and the uninsured.

Clearly, consumer advocates place their priority on preserving service. The governor and care management leaders place a priority on cost containment. These would appear to be opposing and irreconcilable positions. If individuals enrolled in Medicaid plans could join the conversation, would they say that the state is getting value for the money spent? Would they agree that all safety net providers give high-quality care? What kinds of changes would they propose to improve quality? Would their suggestions also lower costs? Medicaid is the current flash point for political and budgetary conflict as the ACA is implemented. In this environment, will changes to Medicaid improve the care received by groups who live with health care inequity?

## HEALTH CARE INEQUITY, SOONERCARE, AND OKLAHOMA'S STRATEGIC COVERAGE INITIATIVE

In 2009, the state government of Oklahoma convened a working group to discuss health care access for either side of the Medicaid income eligibility divide. The product of the group deliberations was the *Oklahoma Strategic Coverage Initiative* (SCI). The SCI contained proposals to meet the access issues of low-wage workers. During the same period, Mathematica evaluated the performance of the Oklahoma Medicaid program.

One core idea unites these reports: minimum health care security. The Executive Summary of the SCI begins with the following description of the health care marketplace reality:

> Over six hundred thousand Oklahomans are without the security of health insurance. In order to create an environment where almost all Oklahomans are insured, such coverage may well require a mandate by state statute. There is no example in any nation, or in any other state, where near universal coverage percentages have been achieved voluntarily. . . . Therefore this Plan recommends that the strategic direction emphasize optimizing enrollments with current programs— then a serious consideration of requiring the individual purchase of health insurance in a fair and equitable manner. An individual mandate should be accompanied by legislation requiring guaranteed issue of lower cost health plans.

The rationale for requiring the individual purchase of health insurance is the need to stabilize financing and standardize benefits on both sides of the Medicaid eligibility barrier:

> When fully funded and operational, the Insure Oklahoma expansions and the Affordable Plans will provide all Oklahomans with the opportunity to enroll in a health plan at reasonable cost.

The ACA calls this policy *individual responsibility* (Title I). The popular press calls it the *individual mandate*. The process leading to this recommendation by the SCI can be traced to Oklahoma's Medicaid cost–control efforts and the beginning of SoonerCare. SoonerCare was a cost-control device to address the widespread dissatisfaction with the quality of the state's Medicaid program. To begin the development of SoonerCare, the Oklahoma legislature created the Oklahoma Health Care Authority (OHCA). This state agency had one mission: it was tasked with converting the state's fee-for-service Medicaid program into a primarily managed-care program. Fee-for-service is easy to understand—every task can be used to generate a separate bill. Managed care is more complex. Managed care—the opposite of fee-for-service—encourages the application of health care as an integrated unit. Maternity care, for example, under fee-for-service can be fractured into a series of separate bills for office visits, lab tests, managing the birth, and a checkup six weeks after the birth. Maternity care in a managed environment would have the same elements.

The pricing, however, would be a comprehensive estimate with no additional billing for extra visits. Women who needed less intensive monitoring would not get a reduction in cost, and women who needed more would not be charged for extra visits. Every mother gets what she needs. All mothers are supported from a common fund. A maternity episode that might end with a vaginal delivery of a healthy baby by a healthy woman is one flat rate. The transition from fee-for-service to managed care was implemented over a 10-year window, resulting in SoonerCare. The evolution of SoonerCare shows the complex web of finance, policy, and politics, creating health care inequity among low-income Oklahomans. The history referenced in this chapter is derived from the SoonerCare report by Mathematica. In this chapter, SoonerCare refers to Medicaid. The SCI refers to employer-sponsored insurance for low-wage workers who are not eligible for SoonerCare.

The SCI was the culmination of a two-year consultation between OHCA, Oklahoma Insurance Department, Oklahoma Health Insurers, and the senior executives of 27 of Oklahoma's largest private sector employers. The sizes of these employers were defined by the numbers in each company's workforce. The language in the preamble to the SCI reflects a centrist political view:

> The proper role of government, on health care and elsewhere, is neither to let broken markets run amok, nor replace the market with bureaucratic mechanisms that set prices and allocate resources. Rather, government's primary role should be to improve the market's ground rules in order to decentralize decision making, spur innovation, reward efficiency, and respect personal choice.

The SCI articulates five strategies:

- Maximizing current opportunity: testing current policy first.
- The affordable (basic) health plans: developing a standard benefit package.
- Generation and application of public revenue: financing health insurance.
- Enrollment strategies: matching individuals with the right program.
- Partnerships: integrating all stakeholders.

Each strategy is intended to be an integrated piece. Once a certain level of progress has been made on these strategies, internal triggers allow each to evolve further. The SCI targets both uninsured persons who are ineligible for SoonerCare as well as their employers. Although it is not explicitly stated, these strategies attack health care inequity by pairing Medicaid policy with employer-sponsored insurance. In 2011, the history surrounding the impact of the SCI on inequity in Oklahoma is still being written. In a November 2011 post on the Oklahoma Policy Blog (OK blog, http:// okpolicy.org/blog/healthcare/employers-better-off-keeping-workers-coverage-under-new-health-law-oklahoma-study-shows), employers are advised that it is better to offer workers' coverage under the ACA. To quote:

> The federal tax code encouraged employers to provide coverage. Known as the "play or pay provision," the ACA law outlines that large employers with 50 or more employees will be subjected to the following:
>
> Those who do not offer coverage will be fined $2,000 per full time employee;
>
> Those offering unaffordable coverage will be subjected to a fee if the employee receives subsidized coverage through the exchange;
>
> Automatic enrollment of employees into their lowest cost option plan if the employee does not sign up or op-out of the employer's coverage.

Mike Rogers, Health Care Committee chair of the Oklahoma State Chamber of Commerce, has analyzed these options and concludes that it would be significantly more expensive for companies to drop coverage.

## WHO IS AT THE SOONERCARE BOUNDARY?

You will find medical need on either side of the SoonerCare eligibility boundary. The groups are distinguished by their financial resources. Patrons of the Indian Health Service are another source of persons on either side of the SoonerCare boundary. In 2003–2004, OHCA conducted a set of studies on the state's uninsured population. They found that in Oklahoma, health care inequity exists largely for the uninsured—those with an income less than 200 percent of FPL (in 2003 dollars) and persons working for a business with 50 or fewer employees. The state agency, OHCA, reported that: (1) about 20 percent (675,000 persons) of the state's population lacked *any* health insurance, placing Oklahoma's uninsured rate at the ninth highest in the nation; (2) 7 in 10 uninsured people were low-income working adults; (3) only 37 percent of small businesses (with 50 or fewer employees) offered health benefits, compared to 47 percent nationally; and (4) small businesses that did not offer employee health benefits ranked financial assistance and flexibility in benefits as important incentives to do so. OHCA had a limited plan—*Insure Oklahoma.* Insure Oklahoma was the beginning of a plan to cover low-wage workers. Are there uninsured workers who are also ineligible for Insure Oklahoma? Yes. Insure Oklahoma only covers persons working for businesses with 250 or fewer employees, low-income college students aged 19 to 22, and children above the Medicaid eligibility cutoff. In addition, some persons would remain uninsured despite the new health plan because, even with substantial subsidies, they could not afford the premiums. According to the SCI, two groups of Oklahomans had the highest risk of being uninsured and ineligible for SoonerCare. Individuals between 19 and 34 years of age comprised *nearly one-half* of Oklahoma's uninsured. The other group finding affordable insurance difficult to obtain was individuals aged 50 to 64. This near-retirement population was partially retired or fully retired and without employer-sponsored retiree health insurance. Many were self-employed. Preexisting condition limitations and medical underwriting restrictions for this age group caused coverage to be unaffordable or unavailable.

Most people agree that it is morally correct to care for the medically needy. Financing this care is another matter. Financing SoonerCare was the main challenge facing Oklahoma when Brad Henry, the newly elected Democratic governor, took office in January 2003. The state was still suffering from revenue shortfalls. SoonerCare enrollment was continuing to grow. The OHCA took additional steps to control costs in early 2003 by eliminating dental services, reducing the number of covered hospital days, and reducing the number of prescription drugs paid per month for adults. As in many states, Oklahoma financed SoonerCare by cobbling together revenue from tobacco taxes, savings from Medicaid-managed care, and general state revenues. Limitations on financing sources to the SoonerCare or Medicaid population prevent Oklahoma—and all other states—from capitalizing on the revenues from other health insurance sources. Insurance premiums from the Insure Oklahoma program are not included in state health care financing resources. Through employer-sponsored plans, these premiums are used to purchase health care from the same system used by SoonerCare clients. Both SoonerCare and Insure Oklahoma use public money to finance health care. This business model of Medicaid segregates high-cost patients in a pool with structural limitations on financing. In most states, the Medicaid-eligible population contains the highest proportion of persons with complex chronic illnesses. Disability is the criterion for eligibility. By omitting the low-wage workers from Medicaid, states limit a source of revenue and increase the probability that any individual member will use expensive health care. The ACA solves this financing limitation by broadening the pool of available fund and decreasing the intensity of health care use by members through its *individual responsibility* (Section 1501) and *employer requirements* (Section 1513) statutes. Without these two requirements, states like Oklahoma find that adequately financing health care for their low-income citizens is impossible. The only other strategies to control Medicaid costs are fluctuating benefit packages—in particular, hospital stays and covered medications. Fluctuating benefits and changing eligibility standards create uncertainty for persons on either side of the Medicaid barrier. Most states use the twin strategies of fluctuating benefits and shifting income eligibility to control Medicaid spending. These cost-control measures create health care inequity.

## THE STRATEGIC COVERAGE INITIATIVE
## AND THE INDIAN HEALTH SERVICE

According to the 2000 census, the state of Oklahoma is home to 333,000 Native Americans. Like all state residents, some Native Americans work for employers who are eligible for Insure Oklahoma. Native Americans can also be found on both sides of the SoonerCare eligibility barrier. By statute, Native Americans can participate in Medicaid if they meet the other eligibility criteria. In short, Native Americans are subject to the same health care inequities imposed by Medicaid eligibility and low-wage employment. Based on tribal affiliations, many Native Americans in Oklahoma are also eligible to obtain health care through the Indian Health Service. Analyses of health disparities consistently identify that underfunding of the Indian Health Service contributes to health care inequity for Native Americans. Underfunding Indian Health Service also contributes to Oklahoma's SoonerCare fiscal issues. Though Mathematica omitted the Indian Health Service from its evaluation of SoonerCare, the SCI examined the role of the Indian Health Service in revamping the state's approach to persons on both sides of the Medicaid divide. Its recognition, however, was limited to a commentary on inadequate federal funding of the Indian Health Service. Others have argued that underfunding of Indian Health Service is a major contributor to health care inequity among American Indians due its effect on state Medicaid budgets. Oklahoma is one of five states where every county has Indian Health Service facilities. Yet, the Indian Health Service does not provide the same package of health care services in each county. In general, the services provided to any particular community will depend on financial resources (i.e., appropriations and third-party reimbursements), available personnel, and facilities. Indian Health Service has stated that its funding does not allow it to provide all the needed care for eligible Native Americans. As a result, according to American Indian health care organizations, some services are rationed, with the most critical care given first. Indian Health Service regulations require that, when resources or funds are insufficient, the agency must set priorities for both direct and contract health care based on *relative medical need*. In addition, Indian Health Service pharmacies may not include all drugs and medicines needed, although Indian Health Service says its pharmacies will stock most drugs that have proven to be cost effective and beneficial. Indian Health Service shortfalls in medical personnel also contribute to this unevenness in health care delivery. In April 2011, the Oklahoma Indian Health Service had 49 vacant positions. There are critical vacancies that include 11 dentists and hygienists; 12 nurses, nurse practitioners, and physician's assistants. The needed 11 physicians include an orthopedic surgeon. There is also a need for two pharmacists.

During its deliberations, the SoonerCare Initiative group was very aware of the Indian Health Service and its contribution to the pool of uninsured and medically underserved persons in Oklahoma:

> The Oklahoma City Area of the Indian Health Service Region is the most inadequately funded region in the United States. A significant number of Oklahoma's uninsured are American Indians. Achieving equity and parity in the funding of Indian Health Service and the tribal services will significantly help Oklahoma.

The Indian Health Service health care delivery program is not an entitlement under federal law. The Indian Health Service cannot commit funding for services if that funding has not been appropriated. Consequently, the services of the Indian Health Service fluctuate each year based on the annual federal appropriation. This makes the Indian Health Service distinct from Medicare. Entitlement programs like Medicaid and Medicare are statutory obligations of the federal government. The federal government must make payments for any person who meets the legal criteria for eligibility. An entitlement program may be funded through either permanent or annual appropriations, but the program's law requires that Congress appropriate whatever funds are needed. One of the major issues addressed in the Indian Health Service reauthorization bills before Congress is the tension between the choices that must be made under the constraints of a finite annual appropriation. An opposing perspective is the view of many American Indians that their health care services are (or should be) an entitlement and, as such, are the sole responsibility of the federal government under trust or treaty obligations. The duty of the federal government to provide health services to Indian tribes derives from a number of different sources, including negotiated treaties to ceded lands, settlements, agreements, and legislation. The principal legislation authorizing federal funds for health services to American Indians is the Snyder Act of 1921. Following the Snyder Act, Congress created a patchwork process for transferring the responsibility of overseeing health programs to tribal governments in 1975. Disputed fiscal responsibility forms the basis for health care inequity in the Indian Health Service delivery system. The inequity intensifies segregation within the Indian Health Service. Facilities that provide care through the Indian Health Service cannot serve patients with private insurance plans. Their ability to garner revenue from sources outside of the Indian Health Service appropriation is blocked. For example, if the closest facility in a rural area is operated by the Indian Health Service, no one else can use it. This limitation in revenue sources starves the facility for the capital necessary for technology and infrastructural upgrades.

The ACA made major amendments to the existing law governing Indian Health Service—the Indian Self-Determination and Education Assistance Act of 1975—by promoting a policy of desegregation. The law updates policy regarding collection of reimbursements from Medicare, Medicaid, and CHIP by Indian Health Service facilities. The changes improve access to capital for doing needed upgrades of Indian Health Service facilities. The ACA contains a provision allowing tribal organizations to purchase coverage for their employees from the Federal Employees Health Benefits Program. This provides for improved insurance coverage at a lower price for the employees of related projects. The ACA also allows tribes and tribal organizations to purchase insurance coverage for Indian Health Service beneficiaries. This means American Indians can purchase supplemental health insurance—just as Medicare beneficiaries have been able to do. ACA authorizes the Indian Health Service to offer hospice, assisted living, long-term care, and community-based services to homebound persons. These benefits have been available under Medicaid for years and are considered an essential part of quality health care. These changes have direct implications for SoonerCare and quality of care for Indians outside and within the Oklahoma Indian Health Service.

## HEALTH CARE INEQUITY AND LONG-TERM CARE SERVICES

Access to long-term care and custodial services is the final piece of the Medicaid and health care inequity story. Medicaid is the number one payer for long-term services and supports in the United States for persons with disabilities in all age groups. Many Americans mistakenly believe that these services are a part of Medicare. There are private insurance policies available, but their monthly premiums are beyond the reach of many. To control spending, each state defines the package of Medicaid-supported long-term services. This has created a crazy quilt of regulations, controls, and operators that vary from state to state. As with other Medicaid plans, long-term services require states to balance their budgets by altering the fund set aside for these benefits. Over the past 10 years, all states have seen an increase in the demand for long-term services. Part of the growth in the population needing Medicaid services is due to successful treatment by health care providers. Health care has increased the number of persons with complex chronic illness and disability by improving survival—individuals who would have died now live for years, needing assistance with personal care, mobility, and cognitive tasks. Modern medicine's ability to prevent disablement does not match its ability to prevent death. Other sections of the ACA recognize the need for better prevention and treatments to restore functional independence. This topic is worthy of discussion, but it is beyond the scope of this chapter. If present trends continue, every life will eventually need the type of long-term care services supported by Medicaid. One can understand the diversity of the population requiring long-term services from the story told by Georgia's mom:

When Georgia was born, I was told that she would not live beyond the first forty eight hours. I would not accept that . . . so I prayed and prayed and . . . she did not die. As time went by, I knew that I was traveling a different road with this child when compared to my four others. It was not one that I would have chosen but there I was. Our family was able to travel this road with state support. . . . It says in Proverbs 17:17 "A friend loveth for all times, and a brother is born for adversity." We were able to care for Georgia all these years because my husband and I had help from her brothers, sisters, and friends. In return, she gave us all a perspective on her alternate road.

A diverse population of individuals requires long-term care services and supports in the United States. Fifty-five percent are elderly, 27 percent are people under the age of 65 with physical disabilities, 15 percent are people with developmental disabilities, and 3 percent are people with chronic mental illness. More than half of these individuals receive services as residents in the community. Some of the services are delivered in their homes. The remainder requires residential care in an institution. Residential care is the most expensive part of Medicaid. In the United States, Medicaid-supported residential care cost states a total of 69 billion dollars. Community-based care serves a larger portion of persons at a significantly lower cost—35 billion dollars for almost 70 percent of this population. We know very little about health care inequity and long-term care.

Medicaid support of long-term services forms a foundation for millions of families like Georgia's across the United States. However, the largest group receiving long-term support is frail elders. In policy circles, these individuals are referred to as *dual eligibles*. Dual eligibles are impoverished individuals who qualify for both the Medicare and the Medicaid programs. Dual eligibles receive their health care services through the Medicare program, while the Medicaid program pays for services and supports not covered by Medicare. These include long-term nursing home stays and physician and hospital co-pays. Frail is another term used to describe this population. Dual eligibles are more likely to have multiple medical problems. In each state, a large portion of Medicaid funds are spent for the care of dual eligibles. Although they are 18 percent of the Medicaid population, dual eligibles account for 46 percent of Medicaid spending. There are currently nine million dual eligibles in the United States. Dual eligibles are disproportionately sicker and are disproportionately members of minority groups when compared to other groups within state Medicaid. Mental illness is an important component of the increased medical needs of this group. Dual eligibles residing in nursing homes are the sickest subset of all public program beneficiaries. The fiscal issues surrounding dual eligibles are best viewed from a state level. For example, there were more than 95,000 dually eligible persons enrolled in Medicaid in Kentucky during 2009. Almost 16 percent of these Medicaid members required nursing home care at an average cost of almost 7,000 dollars per month to the state. Susan Reinhardt of the American Association of

Retired Persons (AARP) described the relationship between disability and Medicaid in the following way:

> Disability . . . can strike at any age. The resulting need for long-term services often takes individuals and their families by surprise. . . . Across the United States, family members and other unpaid caregivers provide most of the services to help people with disabilities remain at home. . . . Public programs that provide assistance for the disabled are uncoordinated, confusing, and underfunded. People are required to impoverish themselves to become eligible. . . . Over the next few years, the United States in effect will choose to create a nationwide, high performing system of long-term services or we can abandon that goal.

Persons who are limited in their ability to live independently experience health care inequities. As they age, health disparities become more prevalent. ACA continues programs designed to help states rebalance the funds available in Medicaid. One program is called *Money Follows the Person* (MFP). MFP capitalizes on the idea that some institutional residents are able and willing to return to living in the community. Federal funds are given to states to support participants during or after a one-year transition period. To get the funds, states need to enact laws to change their policies. Many of these policies require residents in an institution to attain eligibility for Medicaid support. This requirement is particularly problematic for newly disabled adults. Some of these changes include setting aside the residential requirement. Some states already have experimental programs lowering the residential requirement. The numbers of persons who are allowed to participate are limited. MFP funds are available to states that increase the number of participants. Federal funds are also available for states wanting to start new consumer direction options in long-term care through its *Community First Choice Option*. Eligibility is limited to residents in place for six or more months. Transition is most difficult for frail older adults. Debra Lipson, Noelle Denny-Brown, and Susan R. Williams of Mathematica report that fewer eligible persons were actually transitioned during the first few years of the program. There were also fewer transitions than expected.

The ACA contains policies to encourage improvements in our current system of long-term services and support programs. As this chapter is being written, states are hoping for economic recovery while implementing these programs. Medicaid-supported long-term services operate *in parallel* with Medicaid's health insurance function described in the early part of this chapter. In essence, Medicaid is a public insurance plan for the most impoverished, medically vulnerable, and politically unconnected segment of the U.S. population. Because of low birth rates and increased life expectancy among all racial and ethnic groups, the population of the United States is aging rapidly.

Consequently, the United States is struggling with the increasing long-term services burden brought on by the economic and medical needs of this growing population. With every policy change in health care, there is both potential risk and benefit for existing patterns of health care inequity. The equation balancing risk and benefit is not limited to an individual person. While some elders live alone, others receive long-term services from family. Some economists have described caregiving as an intergenerational transfer of wealth from young to old. Others have called the caregivers the *sandwich generation*. Researchers have identified lost wages, little or no retirement savings, and decreased personal health as additional costs of long-term services. To understand the risk, we must have a clear view of the population being served and the extended costs. The nation must be clear about its goals and commitments to these vulnerable citizens.

A country's approach to the problem of old age dependency is structured by its culture, history, and economy. In a racially and culturally diverse nation like the United States, official policy regarding the care of the elderly is not based on a common set of norms concerning the family's role in the care of its oldest members. In the United States, state and federal governments assume the major responsibility for the elderly through Medicare and Medicaid. There is a delicate balance between long-term services utilizing family caregivers while at the same time easing the burden placed on them. Ronald Angel and Jacqueline Angel (1997) make this argument:

> Policies [should] support a system that does not have poor black and Hispanic families shouldering the majority of care giving for aging relatives simply because family is available, while the more affluent non-Hispanic whites receive high quality institutional care.

Where the ACA policy will take current patterns of caregiving is uncertain. At this time, however, it is clear that the ACA involves a shift away from institutionalized care toward personalized care delivered within the home. Will the move toward home-based services increase access? Prior to the ACA, there was clear evidence that persons of color, persons with limited resources, and legal immigrants encounter barriers when accessing Medicaid-supported services. It will be a number of years before we accumulate enough experience to understand the impact of these new policies. On October 14, 2011, the Secretary of Health and Human Services, Kathleen Sebelius, announced that the Community Living Assistance Services and Supports Act portion of the ACA would not be implemented. The CLASS Act, as it was known, was designed to be a long-term care insurance program. The reasons behind dismantlement of the program have not been released.

## POLICIES

The ACA includes a provision to address the needs of people living with disabilities and elderly individuals who require long-term care. This provision extends the *MFP Rebalancing Demonstration Program* through 2020. The original program was authorized by Congress in Section 6071 of the Deficit Reduction Act of 2005. It helps states shift Medicaid's long-term care spending from institutionalized care to community-based services. MFP provides the states with resources and program flexibilities to remove barriers and increase access to community supports that promote independent living. MFP is also designed to help the transition of Medicaid enrollees from institutions to the community. It also reduces the length of time a person is required to reside in an institutional setting before they are eligible to participate in this program. Previously, the requirement was at least six months. At present, the requirement is at least 90 consecutive days. The policy has been in the field for at least 12 months at the time of this writing. In July 2010, nearly 9,000 individuals have been transitioned back to the community and another 4,000 transitions are currently in progress. Community First Choice Option is a program to provide community-based attendant supports and services to individuals with disabilities who require institutional level of care. The ACA gives states an enhanced federal matching rate of six percentage points for reimbursable expenses in the program. This match rate will end after five years.

## CURRENT ENVIRONMENT IN THE STATES

The current economic environment has the potential to increase health care inequities. As states grapple with the deepest budget shortfalls since the depression of 1929, they must also plan for implementation of an expansion of Medicaid health care insurance coverage of childless adults with incomes less than 133 percent of poverty level. To encourage states to take on this additional responsibility, the federal government has offered enhanced matching funds. However, states can receive these funds only if they do not restrict Medicaid eligibility standards. Medicaid serves a population that cannot accommodate increases in premiums. During the period of implementation—before anticipated savings appear—restriction of services is the only option available to balance state budgets. In 2010, nine states put into action restrictions such as reduced personal service hour or respite hour limits (Kansas, New Mexico), increased stringency of medical necessity definition (New Jersey, Colorado, Florida, North Carolina), reduced available budget for subsets of enrollees (Minnesota, Louisiana), and decreased the number of aged and disabled slots to 2007–2008 levels (South Carolina). In 2011, six more states authorized restrictions. Some states instituted caps on the numbers of participants in programs (Missouri—Adult Day Service; South Carolina—HIV/AIDS), caps on the numbers served in long-term care programs (New Hampshire), prior authorization requirements (Iowa), and reduction in respite care hours (Virginia). North Carolina has decided to eliminate community support services. The structure and content of long-term services is an evolving story. Each of these actions has a direct impact on individuals, families, and communities caring for disabled persons and frail elders.

## SUMMARY

Reform of long-term services was included in the ACA. As with the other parts of this legislation, the reform comes with considerable risk. There are examples in recent U.S. history that provide guidance as we roll out these new delivery systems. Events during the 20 years prior to the Mental Health Systems Act of 1980 illustrate the challenges that await the ACA—Medicaid reform. This period is eerily similar to the present in that the United States was at war (Vietnam) and had a fiscal crisis in the 1970s. This combination led to underfunding of new state-level facilities—Community Mental Health Centers. An unbalanced consideration of patient and family issues added to the difficulty of the implementation process. Release of medically needy persons into communities without personnel or resources created law-enforcement issues. Eventually, Community Mental Health Centers across the United States closed.

There was a transition in political power during the implementation of the Mental Health Systems Act of 1980 (Public Law, 96-398). President

James Earl Carter was succeeded by President Ronald Reagan. The law signed by Jimmy Carter was rescinded by Ronald Reagan. Its rescission abdicated federal responsibility and left the states holding the financial responsibility. Mental health professionals were also concerned because patients were not receiving adequate care. An estimate of the homeless population in the 1980s ranged from 250,000 to 500,000. Of these, approximately one-third had a diagnosis of mental illness. In many cases, mentally ill patients were arrested for vagrancy and other minor infractions and were processed by the criminal justice system. MFP supports transition from institution to community. Early reports from the MFP roll-out have already identified housing as a barrier to full use of the new program. Will we see a return to the graying of the homeless population if ACA Medicaid provisions are rescinded?

The ACA emphasizes policies that promote the insurance model and services provided by private sector companies. One risk all communities face with the Community First Choice Option and the MFP is a loss of nursing home beds. In mental health reform history, the combination of Community Health Centers and an emphasis on private sector care led to a decline in publically funded inpatient beds. This problem persists today. The number of beds available to the mentally ill in Washington State dropped 14 percent between 2000 and 2005. Most of this decline was due to cuts in public hospitals. Over time, the change in availability of nursing home beds is something that advocacy groups will need to monitor. With a growth in insurance, there is a potential for profit in the insurance sector and in the provision of home-based services. There is also a real risk of fraud. Fraud and this vulnerable population is a separate topic for discussion in a later chapter. The political challenge facing Medicaid reform is the philosophical difference between social conservatives and those who favor the idea of a social safety net. The 2012 election is an important and risky time for ACA Medicaid reform. The outcome of this election will have a major impact on the current patterns of health care inequity and Medicaid's role in changing those patterns.

## BIBLIOGRAPHY

Agency for Healthcare Research and Quality. "Consumer Assessment of Healthcare Providers and Systems (CAHPS) Surveys and Tools to Advance Patient-Centered Care," http://www.cahps.ahrq.gov/default.asp.

Angel, Ronald, and Jacqueline Angel. *Who Will Care for Us?: Aging and Long-Term Care in Multicultural America*. New York: NYU Press, 1997.

Bachrach, Deborah. "Medicaid Payment Reform: What Policymakers Need to Know About Federal Law." *Policy Brief*, 13, Center for Health Care Strategies, Inc., 2010.

Bachrach, Deborah. "Payment Reform: Creating a Sustainable Future for Medicaid." *Policy Brief*, 14, Center for Health Care Strategies, Inc., 2010.

Bagchi, Ann D., Dominick Esposito, and James M. Verdier. "Prescription Drug Use and Expenditures among Dually Eligible Beneficiaries." *Health Care Financing Review* 28, no. 4 (2007): 14, http://www.mathematica-mpr.com/publications/pdfs/prescriptiondrug.pdf.

Barker, Robert L. *The Social Work Dictionary*. 5th ed. Washington, DC: National Association of Social Workers, 1995.

Barker, David W., Joseph J. Sudano, Ramon Durazo-Arvizu, Joseph Feinglass, Whitney P. Witt, and Jason Thompson. "Health Insurance Coverage and the Risk of Decline in Overall Health and Death among the near Elderly, 1992–2002." *Medical Care* 44, no. 3 (2006): 277–82.

Becker, Alvin, and Herbert C. Schulberg. "Phasing out State Hospitals: A Psychiatric Dilemma." *New England Journal of Medicine* 294, no. 5 (1976): 255–61, http://www.ncbi.nlm.nih.gov/pubmed/811988.

Berkowitz, Edward. "Medicare and Medicaid: The Past as Prologue." *Health Care Financing Review* 27, no. 2 (2005): 11–23.

Clarke, Arthur C. *The Nine Billion Names of God: The Best Short Stories*. New York, NY: Signet/ New American Library, 1996. Paperback 978045 1083814.

Coburn, Tom, and Dennis Smith. "Expanding the Medicaid Status Quo Is Not Health Reform." *National Review Online,* 2009. Published electronically October 19, 2009, http://www.nationalreview.com/critical-condition/48048/expanding-medicaid-status-quo-not-health-reform/tom-coburn.

Conway, Craig A. "Indian Health Care Improvement Act Made Permanent by Health Care Reform Legislation." *Health Law Perspectives,* 2010. Published electronically April 2010, http://www.law.uh.edu/healthlaw/perspectives/2010/%28CC%29%20IHCIA.pdf.

Coughlin, Teresa, Timothy Waidmann, and Molly O'Malley Watts. "Where Does the Burden Lie? Medicaid and Medicare Spending for Dual Eligible Beneficiaries." *Kaiser Commission on Medicaid and the Uninsured.* Washington, DC: Kaiser Family Foundation, 2009.

"Cuomo, Andrew." http://www.governor.ny.gov.Dear, Michael J., and Jennifer R. Wolch. *Landscapes of Despair: From Deinstitutionalization to Homelessness.* 1st ed. Princeton, NJ: Princeton University Press, 1987.

Dicken, John E., Will Simerl, Rashmi Agarwal, Karen Howard, Julian Klazkin, Alexis MacDonald, Daniel Ries, Timothy Walker, and Michael Zose. "Medicaid Outpatient Prescription Drugs: Second Quarter 2008 Federal Upper Limits for Reimbursement Compared with Average Retail Pharmacy Acquisition Costs." Government Accountability Office, 2009.

Gardner, Amanda. "Few Support 'Individual Mandate' in Health Care Reform Law, Poll Finds." *Bloomberg Businessweek,* 2011. Published electronically March 1, 2011, http://www.businessweek.com/lifestyle/content/healthday/650359.html.

Goodman, David C. "Unwarranted Variation Next Term in Pediatric Medical Care." *Pediatric Clinics of North America* 56, no. 4 (2009): 745–55.

Goodman, David C., and Elliott S. Fisher. "Physician Workforce Crisis? Wrong Diagnosis, Wrong Prescription." *New England Journal of Medicine* 358 (2008): 1658–61, http://www.nejm.org/doi/full/10.1056/NEJMp0800 319.

Government Accountability Office. "Health Care: Approaches to Address Racial and Ethnic Disparities. Briefing for Congressional Staff of Senator Bill Frist, Majority Leader, United States Senate," edited by Government Accountability Office, Washington, DC, 2003.

"Governor Cuomo Accepts Recommendations from the Medicaid Redesign Team," http://www.governor.ny.gov/press/022411cuomoaccepts_medicaid redesignteam.

Gruber, Jonathan. "Covering the Uninsured in the United States." *Journal of Economic Literature* 46, no. 3 (2008): 571–606.

Henry, Brad. "Fy-2005 Executive Budget Historical Document," edited by Office of State Finance, Oklahoma City, 2004.

Hollingsworth, Ellen Jane. "Falling through the Cracks: Care of the Chronically Mentally Ill in the United States, Germany, and the United Kingdom." In *Care of the Chronically and Severely Ill: Comparative Social Policies*, edited by Ellen Jane Hollingsworth and J. Rogers Hollingsworth. New York, NY: Aldine de Gruyter, 1994.

Irvin, C., D. Lipson, S. Simon, A. Wenzlow, and J. Ballou. "Money Follows the Person 2009 Annual Evaluation Report," 120, Mathematica Policy Research, Inc., 2010.

"Issue Brief # 7952: Medicaid and Children's Health Insurance Program Provisions in the New Health Reform Law." Focus on Health Reform, 12, Washington, DC, 2010.

Jencks, Cristopher. *The Homeless*. Cambridge, MA: Harvard University Press, 1995.

Kaiser Family Foundation. "Women's Access to Care: A State-Level Analysis of Key Health Policies." Kaiser Family Foundation and National Women's Law Center, 2003.

Kaiser Family Foundation. "Financing New Medicaid Coverage under Health Reform: The Role of the Federal Government and States," 6, Washington, DC, 2010.

Kaiser Family Foundation. "Medicaid Home and Community-Based Service Programs: Data Update," edited by Kaiser Commission on Medicaid and the Uninsured, 2011.

Kaiser Family Foundation. "Money Follows the Person: A 2010 Snapshot." Kaiser Commission on Medicaid and the Uninsured, Washington, DC, 2011.

Kassel, Lara. "Medicaid Matters New York," http://www.medicaidmattersny.org/.

Kaye, H. Stephen, Charlene Harrington, and Mitchell P. LaPlante. "Long-term Care: Who Gets It, Who Provides It, Who Pays, and How Much?" *Health Affairs* 29, no. 1 (2010): 12, http://content.healthaffairs.org/content/29/1/11. abstract.

Kuschell-Haworth, Holly T. "Jumping through Hoops: Traditional Healers and the Indian Health Care Improvement." *DePaul Journal of Health Care Law* 2 (1999): 843–60.

De Leonardis, Ota, and Diana Mauri. "From Deinstitutionalization to the Social Enterprise." *Social Policy* 23, no. 2 (1992): 50–54, http://www.ncbi.nlm. nih.gov/pubmed/10123892.

Miles, Toni P. "Impact of Reform in the United States Health Care Markets on Health Disparities." *Public Policy and Aging Report* 19, no. 4 (2010): 15–18.

Milligan, Chuck. "Reshaping Medicaid." Paper presented at the National Governors Association (NGA) State Summit on Health Reform, Washington, DC, 2010.

National Committee for Quality Assurance. "Health Plan Report Card," http:// reportcard.ncqa.org/plan/external/.

Oklahoma Department of Insurance. "Oklahoma Strategic Plan," edited by Oklahoma State Coverage Initiative, 25, 2009.

Oklahoma State Department of Health. "Behavioral Risk Factor Surveillance System (BRFSS) 2007 Annual Report." Oklahoma City, OK, 2007.

Oklahoma State Department of Health. "Oklahoma Behavioral Risk Factor Surveillance System 58, 73117." Oklahoma City, OK, 2007.

Patient Protection and Affordable Care Act. Public Law 111–148. March 23, 2010.

Podrazik, Mark, and Anne Winter. "Independent Evaluation of the Insure Oklahoma Program," 129, Burns and Associates, Inc., Phoenix, AZ, 2008.

Pries, J.L., C. Cook, S.P. Burch, and C.R. Cantrell. "Racial Differences in Quality Care Measures, Medication Adherence, Health Care Costs, and Utilization with Common Chronic Diseases in a 9-State Medicaid Population." Paper presented at the American Public Health Association 137th annual meeting, Philadelphia, 2009.

Quesnel-Vallée, Amélie. "Is It Really Worse to Have Public Health Insurance Than to Have No Insurance at All? Health Insurance and Adult Health in the United States." *Journal of Health and Social Behavior* 45, no. 4 (2004): 376–92.

Rachlin, Stephen. "With Liberty and Psychosis for All." *Psychiatric Quarterly* 48, no. 3 (1974): 410–20.

Rachlin, Stephen, Alvin Pam, and Janet Milton. "Civil Liberties Versus Involuntary Hospitalization." *American Journal of Psychiatry* 132, no. 2 (1974): 189–92.

Ranji, Usha, Alina Salganicoff, Alexandra M. Stewart, Marisa Cox, and Lauren Doamekpor. State Medicaid Coverage of Perinatal Services: Summary of State Survey Findings, Kaiser Family Foundation and The George Washington University School of Public Health and Health Services, Washington, DC, 2009.

Rebhun, Uzi, and Adi Raveh. "The Spatial Distribution of Quality of Life in the United States and Interstate Migration, 1965–1970 and 1985–1990." *Social Indicators Research* 78, no. 1 (2006): 137–78.

Reinhard, Susan C., Enid Kassner, and Ari Houser. "How the ACA Can Help Move States toward a High Performing System of Long-Term Services and Supports." *Health Affairs* 30, no. 3 (2011): 447–53.

Revelle, Randy. "Inpatient Mental Health: Community Hospitals in Crisis," 12, Washington State Hospital Association, Seattle, WA, 2005.

Rossi, Peter H. *Down and out in America: The Origins of Homelessness*. Chicago, IL: University of Chicago Press, 1989.

Saathoff, Gregory B., Jorge A. Cortina, Ronald Jacobson, and C. Knight Aldrich. "Mortality among Elderly Patients Discharged from a State Hospital." *Hospital & Community Psychiatry* 43, no. 3 (1992): 280–81.

Shapiro, Lila. "Kyl: 'I Don't Need Maternity Care' So Employers Shouldn't Be Required to Provide It." *Huffington Post,* 2009, http://www.huffingtonpost.com/2009/09/25/kyl-i-dont-need-maternity_n_300367.html.

Shwed, Harvey J. "Protecting the Rights of the Mentally Ill." *American Bar Association Journal* 64 (1978): 564–67.

Shwed, Harvey J. "Social Policy and the Rights of the Mentally Ill: Time for Re-Examination." *Journal of Health Politics, Policy and Law* 5, no. 2 (1980): 193–98.

Smedley, Brian D. "Moving beyond Access: Achieving Equity in State Health Care Reform." *Health Affairs* 27, no. 2 (2008): 447–55.

Smith, Vernon K., Kathleen Gifford, Eileen Ellis, Robin Rudowitz, and Laura Synder. "Report #8105 Hoping for Economic Recovery, Preparing for Health Reform: A Look at Medicaid Spending, Coverage and Policy Trends." In *Kaiser Commission on Medicaid and the Uninsured*. Washington, DC: The Henry J. Kaiser Family Foundation, 2010.

Talbott, John A. "The Care of the Chronically Mentally Ill, Deinstitutionalization, and Homelessness in the United States." *Psychiatric Humanarica* 7 (1992): 615–26.

Thomas, Alexander. "Ronald Reagan and the Commitment of the Mentally Ill: Capital, Interest Groups, and the Eclipse of Social Policy." *Electronic Journal of Sociology* 3, (1998), http://www.sociology.org/content/vol003.004/thomas.html.

Udom, Nduka U., and Charles L. Betley. "Effects of Maternity-Stay Legislation on 'Drive-through Deliveries.'" *Health Affairs* 17, no. 5 (1998): 208–15.

U.S. Bureau of Labor Statistics. "On Benefits by Wage Level." Program Perspectives, 2010.

U.S. Congress, Public Health Service Act. Public Law 78–409, 58. July 1, 1944.

U.S. Department of Health and Human Services. "Indian Health Care Improvement Act Made Permanent." Health and Human Services, http://www.hhs.gov/news/press/2010pres/03/20100326a.html.

Verdier, James M., Margaret Colby, Debra Lipson, Samuel Simon, Christal Stone, Thomas Bell, Vivian Byrd, Mindy Lipson, and Victoria Pérez. "SoonerCare 1115 Waiver Evaluation: Final Report." Mathematica Policy Research, Inc, Washington, DC, 2009.

Willie, Lynette. "America Reaffirms Health Care for Indian Country." National Indian Health Board, http://www.nihb.org/docs/03212010/PR-03.21.10%20FINAL.pdf.

Worley, Nancy K., and Barbara J. Lowery. "Deinstitutionalization: Could It Have Been Better for Patients." *Archives of Psychiatric Nursing* 2, no. 3 (1988): 126–33.

Wright, James D. *Address Unknown: The Homeless in America.* Hawthorne, NY: Aldine de Gruyter, 1989.

Zaman, Obaid S., Linda C. Cummings, and Sari Siegel Spieler. "America's Public Hospitals and Health Systems 2008." National Association of Public Hospitals and Health Systems, 2010.

# CHAPTER 3

## Quality, Disparity, and Title III

There are 10 titles in the Affordable Care Act (ACA). Title III— *Improving the quality and efficiency of health care*—has had little discussion. Its dense language does not generate the sound bites of 15 and 30 seconds favored by the media. Policy wonks like to debate this title and its potential to make the delivery system better. The impact of Title III on disparity is not on anyone's list of topics for conversation. Even the most dedicated policy analyst gets lost in the language of quality. Words like *quality, safety,* and *access* get tossed around. What do these ideas look like in practice? Quality is like mom and apple pie. Who could be against that? The idea of poor quality care has deep roots in the history of American medical apartheid. Byrd and Clayton provide extensive documentation that African Americans were purposefully injured by the physicians they had to rely on for care. The experience of other groups with medical research is another dark chapter in the U.S. health care. With each episode of unethical medical research, there was an idea that some groups in American society—prisoners, immigrants, non-English speakers, workers—were not worthy of the highest level of health care. In 1966, Henry K. Beecher published an article in the New England Journal of Medicine describing the routine nature of human subject experimentation in U.S. medicine and its unethical practices. His work led to the regulations we now have in place for the protection of research participants. Title 45 Code of Federal Regulation Part 46 defines categories of protection. Biomedical research is necessary for the development of safe and effective treatments. The participant must be a willing participant and that consent is not based on deceptive practices. In short, the promise of treatment cannot be the sole basis for recruitment.

Health care inequity is a different issue. Medical research regulations did not and could not contend with the idea that one social class (moneyed, educated) delivers health care to all other social classes. Bear in mind, the broad regulation of medical research only began in the 1970s with the Belmont Report. The idea that health care providers will be held accountable for the standard of quality only began to take shape in the 1990s with the work of the National Quality Care Forum. Tools used in clinical practice to measure quality of care are available through the National Quality Measures Clearinghouse. The clearinghouse is a public resource for evidence-based quality measures. The idea that poor quality care contributes to health disparities is still in its developmental stages for researchers and practitioners. Inequity is still a separate idea from quality. For example, ACA Title III Section 3001 describes the Hospital Value Based Purchasing Program. In the text, hospitals are required to document race, ethnicity, and other characteristics of patients. The goal is to measure differences in treatment for different groups. For the first time in U.S. history, we will be able to identify hospitals that provide poor quality care *within their walls* to different groups. Not only does Title III provide data to *see* poor quality, it also provides remedies to change the practices of providers. Practice change is linked to payment. In general, quality and inequity do not get the attention they deserve. Discussions of the two issues are obscured by policy language.

The complexity of the health care delivery system leads to obsessive specialization among policy analysts. Policy analysts with an interest in hospital access policy and disparity talk about utilization of the emergency department. Policy analysts who have an interest in Medicare and disparity talk about Medicare recipients who are so poor that they are eligible for both Medicare and Medicaid. This group of enrollees is referred to as the dual eligibles or *dualies*. Policy analysts who have an interest in medication costs and disparity talk about the Medicare Prescription Drug Plan (Part D) coverage gap or *donut hole*. If you are in the donut hole, you have to pay the entire cost of your medications. This coverage gap starts at approximately 2,700 dollars. You are wholly responsible for the next 3,453 dollars worth of medication costs. Inappropriate emergency room usage, dual eligibility, and prescription medication costs are three simple examples of disparity. Title III has specific policies to address the disparities caused by each.

Medicare payment played a leading role in opening health care access in the United States. Hospital desegregation, medical care for poor elders, physician training, and fiscal stability for rural health care are all by-products of Medicare legislation. ACA Title III, Subtitle G, Sections 3601 and 3602 define a minimum benefit in Medicare. This title aligns public insurance benefits with the private insurance market benefits in Title I— essential benefits. Section 3601 defines a floor for traditional Medicare benefits at their current level. The quality initiatives in the ACA will generate program savings. The law requires that the savings are reinvested in Medicare as either new benefits or a reduction in premiums. Section 3602 preserves the benefits included in Medicare Advantage Plans. Unlike Section 3601, Section 3602 does not guarantee that Medicare Advantage Plans will cost less. In plain language, Medicare Advantage Plan beneficiaries will pay more for the extra benefits that are included in the Advantage Plans. These benefits include things like eyeglasses, hearing aids, and gym membership (*SilverSneakers*). This change will structure Medicare Advantage Plans to resemble the employer-sponsored plans. Employer-sponsored health insurance plans supply basic outpatient and hospital care. Items such as eyeglasses, dental care, and prescription coverage are extra. Medicare Advantage Plan beneficiaries, like all Medicare enrollees, will continue to have prescription drug insurance. For those who need confirmation of the legislative text, the following is taken verbatim from 42 U.S. Code 1395 and 1395w-21:

## SUBTITLE G—PROTECTING AND IMPROVING GUARANTEED MEDICARE BENEFITS

### SEC. 3601—Protecting and Improving Guaranteed Medicare Benefits

*Protecting Guaranteed Medicare Benefits.*—Nothing in the provisions of, or amendments made by, this Act shall result in a reduction of guaranteed benefits under Title XVIII of the Social Security Act.

*Ensuring that Medicare Savings Benefit the Medicare Program and Medicare Beneficiaries.*—Savings generated for the Medicare program under Title XVII of the Social Security Act under the provisions of, and amendments made by, this Act shall extend the solvency of the Medicare trust funds, reduce Medicare premiums, and other cost-sharing for beneficiaries, and improve or expand guaranteed Medicare benefits and protect access to Medicare providers.

## SEC. 3602—No Cuts in Guaranteed Benefits

Nothing in this Act shall result in the reduction or elimination of any benefits guaranteed by law to participants in Medicare Advantage.

To connect the quality movement and the conversation surrounding disparity, let us use a metaphor about flight. The level of the debate on the topic of *quality* can be (1) very high—50,000 feet, (2) somewhat high—5,000 feet, or (3) skimming across the ground at 5 feet. Quality in health care is experienced at each of these levels. Disparity in health care is measured at all levels. At the five-foot level, persons who cannot obtain timely, appropriate, and effective primary care are the ones who utilize emergency departments, require hospitalizations, and die too soon. Hospitalizations for pulmonary conditions such as asthma and chronic obstructive pulmonary disease are rising and reflect the declining access to care. Getting admitted to the hospital does not guarantee adequate care. Twenty percent of persons return to the hospital soon after discharge because of a complication. These complications could be prevented with careful attention to the process of transition from hospital to home. All patients have the potential to experience a complication after hospital discharge. Many come from health disparity groups. The ACA addresses the problem of quality surrounding hospital discharge in Section 2704. This demonstration project is designed to evaluate programs that integrate care across the transition from hospital to home. Once the program is complete, all hospitals will be required to adopt this process. Program development, evaluation, and integration into practice are the process the ACA recognizes as *quality in health care*. These practices will benefit all patients, not just disparity groups by creating patient-centered care.

By contrast, at 50,000 feet *quality* involves payment strategies used by the public plans—Medicare and Medicaid. The views from five feet and 5,000 feet make the discussion of quality and disparities complicated. To keep things simple, quality advocates tend to focus only on one level. Although advocates are passionate about the issue, there is a tendency to minimize the importance of elements that do not appear at one's own level and to maximize the importance of those that do. Advocates of 50,000 feet emphasize federal programs, federal appropriations, and preservation of federal funding. ACA Section 2602 recognizes a quality of care issue for dual eligible beneficiaries. This section creates a Federal Coordinated Health Care Office for such beneficiaries in the Center for Medicare and Medicaid Services (CMS). This office integrates Medicare and Medicaid benefits by linking federal and state governments. ACA Section 3021 establishes the Centers for Medicare and Medicaid Innovation within the CMS. This office coordinates innovative payment and service delivery models to promote quality and efficiency. It provides the secretary flexibility to pilot and implement an innovative Medicare payment model using a variety of models, including medical homes. Advocates have long recognized that care coordination and rapid transmission of care delivery models lead to quality health care. Will disparity advocates also see a closure in the gap between populations with the advent of a medical home?

Health care equity advocates have struggled with a strategy to measure disparity. Without a measurement, how are you going to know that things are getting better? In its health care quality reports of 2009, the Agency for Healthcare Research and Quality creates an operational definition for health disparities. *Health disparities* refer to gaps in the quality of health and health care across racial (http://en.wikipedia.org/wiki/Race_%28classification_of_human_beings%29), ethnic, and socioeconomic groups. The Health Resources and Services Administration define health disparities as population-specific differences in the presence of disease, health outcomes, or access to health care. With this statistic, health disparities are well documented in minority populations such as African Americans, Native Americans, Asian Americans, and Latinos. When compared to whites, these minority groups have higher incidence of chronic diseases, higher mortality, and poorer health outcomes. Health disparities are also well documented among persons with less than the U.S. median income of 40,000 dollars with less than 12 years of schooling, and low health literacy. How does Title III of the ACA change the way we think, talk about, and work on health care disparities? To illustrate the quality movement and its potential, let us take two big ideas currently under discussion among quality policy wonks. These ideas are *health literacy* and *patient-centered care*.

## HEALTH LITERACY

Front line providers emphasize individual characteristics like *health literacy*. This is an issue most easily seen at the five-foot level. Health literacy is the ability to obtain, process, and understand basic health information and services needed to make appropriate health decisions. Literacy is also required to follow treatment instructions. The Centers for Disease Control and Prevention (CDC) estimate that more than 89 million American adults have limited health literacy skills. People of all ages, races, incomes, and education levels are challenged by this problem. Individuals with limited health literacy incur medical expenses that are up to four times greater than patients with adequate literacy skills, costing the health care system billions of dollars every year.

The solution to the problem of health literacy rests with the training of *health care professionals*. Research supports the idea that improving the communication skills of professionals is an important first step in addressing the problem of health literacy. Skilled communication contributes to quality care by improving:

• Relations between health care professional and their patients.

• Individuals' exposure to, search for, and use of health information.

• Individuals' agreement with clinical recommendations and regimens.

• Education of consumers about access to health care.

It is clear that health literacy enhances the quality care. The key to literacy is becoming a lifelong learner. In the current era, Internet access is the pathway of choice for learning and communication. This is particularly true for knowledge of health care related information. Disparity exists wherever there are barriers to obtaining information and missing communications technology. Regardless of years in school or reading skills, individuals without Internet access will have low levels of health literacy. Hargittai Eszter (2002) published one of the early reports identifying older adults, women, members of racial and ethnic groups, and rural residents as least likely to have the skills required for efficient use of the Internet. These groups are also more likely to live with a disability. Disability is also associated with being older, less educated, and limited financial resources. People with a disability have lower rates of Internet access and lower rates of health literacy. In discussions of communication technologies, the disparity in access to electronic information resources is commonly referred to as the *digital divide* (U.S. Department of Commerce, 1999). The digital divide becomes more critical as the amount and variety of health resources available over the Internet increase. Equitably distributed health communication resources and skills, and a robust communication infrastructure can contribute to the closing of the digital divide and the elimination of health disparities. The ACA does not contain specific provisions to close the digital divide for individuals. It does, however, address the problem of Internet access and electronic health care records for the institutions that serve health disparity groups in Title III, Section 3002—Improvements to the Physician Quality Reporting System.

Even with access to information and services, however, disparities exist because many people lack basic reading skills. Basic reading skills are needed for two essential tasks. One task involves the ability to read and understand materials related to personal health. The other task involves navigating the health care system. Persons who are missing one or both of these tasks will have difficulty accessing health care. This is the path to disparity. People with low literacy are more likely to report poor health. Low literacy leads to an incomplete understanding of one's health problems and treatments. Incomplete understanding of a health problem and its treatment increases the risk for complications and hospitalization. Very low literacy is defined as reading at a grade level two or below average. The average annual health care costs of persons with very low literacy may be four times greater than for the general population. While anyone can have a chronic condition such as asthma, hypertension, or diabetes, low reading skills make management of these conditions challenging.

Although the majority of people with marginal or low literacy are white native-born Americans, changing demographics in the United States will complicate the ability of the health care system to meet this need. Low literacy is a problem among certain racial and ethnic groups, non-English speaking populations, and persons over the age of 65 years. The numbers of persons in these categories are estimated to grow in the coming years. In a safety net hospital setting, a study of patients aged 60 and older found that 81 percent could not read and understand basic materials such as prescription labels and appointments. In an environment with pervasively low literacy, effective communication becomes the responsibility of all health care providers. Improving the communication skills of health care professionals can increase the safety of health care for all groups—not just health disparity groups. Data from the National Assessment of Adult Literacy (NAAL, 2003 in White and Dillow, 2005) show that the tasks required to navigate the health care system require a literacy level beyond *most* patients' capability. In short, health care delivery systems do not pay attention to the effectiveness of their communications. In the National Assessment of Adult Literacy, literacy is based on a rating scale from 0 to 500. A basic level of literacy ranges from 185 to 225. Readers within this performance level can cite two reasons why a person with no symptoms should be screened after reading a clearly written pamphlet. This is the task we demand of men who are considering a Prostate Specific Antigen (PSA) test to screen for prostate cancer. Most discussions begin with the physician giving the patient a pamphlet and asking: *Any questions?* Here is the language used in a pamphlet:

The United States Task Force for Preventive Services recommends [a process called] Shared Decision Making when thinking about the use of the PSA test to screen men without symptoms of prostate disease.

This sentence requires the reading skills of a college freshman. In the health care setting, patients are asked to determine the timing of prescription medication and timing of meals. According to National Assessment of Adult Literacy scores, reading the medication label requires a minimum score of 253. This is considered an intermediate level of literacy. The United States needs a health literacy campaign. Within the context of health disparities, the following story clearly illustrates the challenge. It was told by a colleague who is U.S. born, monolingual, and a family physician:

One day I received a phone call from the hospital that my patient, a forty one year old Hispanic male, was admitted to the medical Intensive Care Unit. I was surprised because I had seen the patient in my office earlier in the week. Aside from newly diagnosed hypertension, he was in excellent physical condition. For appropriate medical reasons, I prescribed a beta blocker to lower his blood pressure. Later, when speaking with his wife, I discovered that he became ill shortly after starting the medication. Upon detailed questioning, I discovered he had taken eleven doses of the blood pressure lowering drug—slowing his heart rate. To my horror, I discovered that my patient, who spoke reasonable English, had difficulty with the English instructions *once daily*. The English word *once* means *eleven* in Spanish.

In the National Assessment of Adult Literacy survey of adults, Medicare beneficiaries were also likely to have lower levels of literacy. The average score ranges from 161 to 222. With this level, almost all beneficiaries would have difficulty with the prostate cancer screening decision task and the blood pressure medication management task described previously. If we are to achieve success with a therapy or testing, health care providers will need to improve their communication skills.

## PATIENT-CENTERED CARE

In its report, the Institute of Medicine describes the connection between quality and disparity in the following language:

[P]atient centeredness is a core component of quality health care. Patient-centeredness is defined as: [H]ealthcare that establishes a partnership among practitioners, patients, and their families (when appropriate) to ensure that decisions respect patients' wants, needs, and preferences and that patients have the education and support they need to make decisions and participate in their own care. . . . [it] encompasses qualities of compassion, empathy, and responsiveness to the needs, values, and expressed preferences of the individual patient. . . . [E]ffective communication between the provider and the patient is often a legal requirement. . . . care is supported by good provider patient communication so that patients' needs and wants are understood and addressed, and patients understand and participate in their own care. This style of care has been shown to improve patients' health and health care. Unfortunately, many barriers exist to good communication. About one third of Americans are not health literate, which means they lack the capacity to obtain, process, and understand basic health information and services needed to make appropriate health decisions. They experience many difficulties, including less preventive care, poorer understanding of their conditions and care, more emergency and inpatient visits, and higher rates of [repeated] hospitalization, lower adherence to medication schedules, and lower participation in medical decision making. Individuals with inadequate health literacy incur higher medical costs and are more likely to have an inefficient mix of service use compared with those with adequate health literacy. Providers also differ in communication proficiency, including varied listening skills and different views from their patients' of symptoms and treatment effectiveness. Additional factors influencing patient-centeredness and provider patient communication include: language barriers, racial and ethnic concordance between the patient and provider, effects of disabilities on patients' health care experiences, and providers' cultural competency.

The present-day quality movement began in earnest during the 1990s. A number of organizations were involved in its development. The Commonwealth Fund, headed by Karen Davis, has promoted its *High Performance Health Care System*. The Robert Wood Johnson Foundation has led an effort to *Align Forces 4 Quality*. In 2006, Gail Warden and Leonard Schaeffer led a team to comprehensively assess reform efforts called *COMPARE*. The National Committee for Quality Assessment has coordinated the development of both Consumer Assessment of Healthcare Providers and

Systems and the Healthcare Effectiveness Data and Information Set. The Consumer Assessment of Healthcare Plans measures satisfaction with insurance. The Healthcare Effectiveness Data and Information Set survey measures appropriateness of care.

The history of the quality movement and relationship to disparities is a work in progress. A seminal paper in 2003 by Galvin and McGlynn made the case for formal measurement of performance. Under the leadership of Carolyn Clancy, MD, the Agency for Healthcare Research and Quality (AHRQ) heads the federal effort to standardize performance. Dr. Clancy has been director of the Agency for Healthcare Research and Quality since 2003. Prior to 2003, she led the Agency for Healthcare Research and Quality's Center for Outcomes and Effectiveness Research. The ACA builds on this movement. For the first time, Medicare payment is tied to patient satisfaction, health care outcomes, and performance. These ideas are not generic terms. Research supported by the Agency for Healthcare Research and Quality has created the specific measures needed to monitor satisfaction, outcomes, and performance. Although the opposition to this movement is not formally documented, anecdotal stories highlight the resistance of health care professionals to the idea that they are a source of poor quality care. Some professionals attribute patient difficulty with management to noncompliance. Others take a paternalistic stance that only a professional knows what is correct. In their writings about quality, Galvin and McGlynn do not discuss disparities. However, they do make a case for the accountability of regulators, insurers, providers, and accrediting organizations to clients. By connecting quality to *all* clients, the quality movement creates a pathway for resolving disparities. This pathway is patient-centered for anyone receiving treatment. To fully illustrate patient-centered care, let us consider the movement for language-appropriate health care.

## LANGUAGE-APPROPRIATE HEALTH CARE

What are the stakes surrounding health care quality and patients with limited English proficiency? According to the U.S. Census Bureau, almost 20 percent of Americans aged five and older speak something other than English at home. The language of choice is Spanish (62%), followed by Indo-European languages (almost 19%), and Asian/Pacific Island languages (15%). Among persons who speak something other than English at home, almost 29 percent of middle-aged and 67 percent older adults are most likely to experience this barrier to health care access. This is also the population most likely to need health care and hospitalization. Perhaps the highest stakes for patients and health care organizations involve advance directives and end-of-life medical expenditures. End-of-life health care accounted for almost one quarter of Medicare spending in 2006. In an analysis of Medicare data, Lauren Nicholas clearly shows that Medicare spending is highest for patients without advanced directives. Advanced directives are a formal approach to making your wishes known about the use of respirators and other therapies during the dying process. In their ideal form, advanced directives are written documents. They are a part of the patient's medical record. These documents are used to communicate for the patient when a patient cannot speak for himself or herself. Castillo and others at the University of California reviewed case law to document the unintended consequences of advance directives on clinical care. They find that poor readability of these laws and limited English proficiency increase the risk for wishes not being honored. Palliative care is an approach that maximizes comfort when cure is not possible. Alexander Smith, Rebecca Sudore, and Eliseo Perez-Stable also make the point that communication barriers between provider and patient can prevent effective palliative care.

To resolve the health care barrier created by language, the Office of Minority Health led a movement to develop national standards. This effort has become known as the Cultural and Linguistic Appropriate Standards. The final report describing Cultural and Linguistic Appropriate Standards was issued in 2001. The idea is simple. A consistent and comprehensive standard for language leads to quality health care. The Cultural and Linguistic Appropriate Standards are potentially one means to correct inequities that currently exist in the provision of care. Cultural and Linguistic Appropriate Standards make care responsive to the individual needs of all patients and consumers. In 2010, only 19 percent of U.S. hospitals met the Cultural and Linguistic Appropriate Standards. This is a dangerous situation for patients.

Cultural and Linguistic Appropriate Standards is a set of 14 standards. Four standards are mandated. The remaining 10 are either guidelines or recommendations. All institutions that receive federal funds must comply with the mandates. Hospitals that serve Medicare and Medicaid beneficiaries, for example, must comply. These four standards are based on Title IV of Civil Rights Act of 1964. The following mandated standards are designed to meet the needs of persons with limited English proficiency:

Standard Four: Health care organizations must offer and provide assistance services, including bilingual staff and interpreter services,

at no cost to each patient and consumer with limited English proficiency at all points of contact, in a timely manner during all hours of
operation.

Standard Five: Health care organizations must provide to patients
and consumers in their preferred language both verbal offers and
written notices informing them of their right to receive language assistance services.

Standard Six: Health care organizations must assure the competence of language assistance provided to limited English proficient
patients and consumers by interpreters and bilingual staff. Family
and friends should not be used to provide interpretation services ex-
cept on request by the patient or consumer.

Standard Seven: Health care organizations must make available
easily understood patient-related materials and post signage in the
languages of the commonly encountered groups and/or groups represented in the service area.

The movement for language-appropriate health care has grown in parallel with two other changes in American society. One trend is the increasing diversity of the U.S. population. In 1999, California's *minority*
population became the majority. Iowa was actively recruiting immigrants
and refugees to meet its workforce shortages. When the federal government begins to actively address a barrier to health care, what does the
process look like? The implementation and the process of development
of Cultural and Linguistic Appropriate Standards in health care provide
clues. The Cultural and Linguistic Appropriate Standards are primarily
directed at health care organizations and individual providers. To initiate a
conversation between government and organizations in the private sector,
an announcement was published in the Federal Register on December 15,
1999, beginning a four-month period of commentary. During that time,
the Office of Minority Health received 413 comments from individuals
and organizations. Some comments were supportive of the proposed standards while others voiced objections. The following comments illustrate
the extremes of opinions and are taken from the Office of Minority Health
final report:

We understand the significance of this activity and the potential that
the standards embody for improving health care outcomes. We share

and support your concern for the need to develop and release clear guidance to plans and other providers as they respond to a rapidly growing, culturally diverse population.

(Anonymous)

[We do] believe that culturally and linguistically appropriate health care services are an area of health care that should be highly regulated. When a guideline or standard is strictly mandated and regulated, all possible opportunities for flexibility and innovation are eliminated. This approach is not in the best interest of the patient or customer needing the service. We believe that health care institutions and other quality businesses will adopt the proposed principals as guidelines to ensure that they provide high quality health care that encompasses the needs of the patient, the patient's family, and the community.

(Mayo Foundation)

Many providers expressed concerns about the cost of compliance with Cultural and Linguistic Appropriate Standards:

unreasonable burden in costs and resources associated with the draft standards . . . if applied literally, they would likely overwhelm most hospital and physician resources—both time and money.

Commentaries from the home health care agencies were concerned about the impact of Cultural and Linguistic Appropriate Standards on their business:

Specifically, Office of Minority Health's proposed Cultural and Linguistic Appropriate Standards would require the financial resources to hire new and additional staff or contract services, as well as to develop new policies and procedures.

Some health care businesses voiced the option that Cultural and Linguistic Appropriate Standards would lead to cost-effective health care"

The National Business Group on Health believes that employer consideration of cultural competence leads to efficient use of health care dollars . . . and can contribute to increased productivity and a reduction in absenteeism and disability. Increased patient compliance and satisfaction can improve health outcomes. As employers respond to an increasingly consumer-driven health system, emphasis on cultural competence and assessment of what services are available and how they're delivered to a diverse workforce will become increasingly important.

The arguments for and against Cultural and Linguistic Appropriate Standards can be summed up in two sentences. Arguments for Cultural and Linguistic Appropriate Standards emphasized the cost of doing nothing and continuing business as usual. Arguments against Cultural and Linguistic Appropriate Standards emphasized the cost of implementing new requirements. Does the ACA build on this process? While there is no explicit reference to Cultural and Linguistic Appropriate Standards, every section describing the development of patient communication materials does explicitly call for linguistically appropriate materials. The use of Cultural and Linguistic Appropriate Standards in health care continues to be an emerging health disparity issue as the U.S. population becomes increasingly diverse.

## A COMMUNITY TACKLES ITS DISPARITIES:
## THE FIVE-FOOT VIEW OF QUALITY

The health care experience is always local. Whether you are ill, injured, or giving birth, treatment is up close and very personal. Although support and guidance from national organizations are helpful, quality changes happen in institutions that maybe just down the street from your house. This final section presents examples of quality-focused undertakings. As of this writing, we do not know the impact these changes have had on local health disparities. We can report on the earliest efforts communities are making to accommodate the quality initiatives of the ACA. First, let us look at a hospital quality initiative. Next, we will discuss the efforts of a community-based organization's efforts to create parity for mental illness care and physical illness care. In each case, the organization leading the way based its efforts on recognized community consensus. For the hospital, there was also a market share competition concern. The work required to improve quality is complex. Each group is experiencing resistance from unexpected quarters. As of this writing, it is not clear that either will be able to continue the process each has initiated. The ACA, however, has distinct provisions to reward these efforts with financing of the involved health care institutions.

## A HOSPITAL QUALITY INITIATIVE: 2011 NATIONAL QUALITY HEALTHCARE AWARD

On March 28, 2011, Norton Healthcare of Louisville, Kentucky, issued the following press release:

> The National Quality Forum (NQF) announced today that Norton Healthcare has been named the recipient of the 2011 NQF National Quality Healthcare Award for its exceptional organizational leadership and innovation to achieve quality improvement. . . . As part of its mission to improve the quality of health care in America, NQF presents this [award] annually to an exemplary . . . organization that has achieved a number of quality focused goals.

Organizations that are eligible for the award include those providing direct patient care and who publically report performance data under voluntary or mandated reporting programs. To get this award, Norton Healthcare has taken tangible steps to achieve measurable patient-focused experience. Norton Healthcare is one of the first health care organizations in the nation to publically report its performance on hundreds of NQF-endorsed quality indicators. A monthly report on the health care system's public website displays side by side numeric results for each hospital in the Norton Healthcare system. The report highlights in green or red any result that is significantly better or worse than the national average. Norton Healthcare has advanced its performance in quality, process, patient safety, and satisfaction. This advance required unification of its hospitals, physician practices, and service lines. If you go to their website, you will see the quality report principles that Norton Healthcare abide by (http://www. nortonhealthcare.com/QualityReport):

- We do not decide what to make public based on how it makes us look.
- We give equal prominence to good and bad results.
- We do not choose which indicators to display. When we have a nationally endorsed list of indicators, we display every indicator on the list.
- We are not the indicator owner. We do not modify indicator definitions, inclusion, or exclusion criteria in any way.

- We correct our internal data only for objective errors. We do not correct data submitted or billed externally unless we also resubmit or rebill the data.
- We display our results even when we disagree with the indicator definition. Unused data never become valid.
- We recognize that we must display and make decisions based upon imperfect data, because until the data are used, no resources will be spent making the data valid.

The Patient Satisfaction portion of Norton's quality report shows patient rating data for six hospitals in their system. CAHPS items—communication with staff, responsiveness of staff, communication with doctors, pain control, quiet around room, and cleanliness of room—are all there. On most measures, Norton Healthcare is near the U.S. average. In October 4, 2011, *noise around the room at night* in Norton hospitals was rated below the U.S. average for all but one of the hospitals. Anyone in the community can return to this website at a future time to track change in patient ratings. This is quality care measurement and communication for hospitals at the five-foot level. As sections of the ACA are implemented, Norton Healthcare will begin reporting gender, race, ethnicity, language, and disability for their patient population. All six hospitals in the Norton Healthcare system are located in and around Jefferson County in Louisville, Kentucky. This county has a population of slightly more than 500,000 persons (2006, U.S. Census Bureau). One-third of the minority population is African American. Less than 2 percent are Hispanic. Six percent speak a language other than English at home. Almost 15 percent are aged 65 and older. Louisville's immigrants are more diverse in their origins than the overall U.S. immigrant population. Latin America accounted for 38 percent of all immigrants in 2004. Fifteen percent of Louisville's immigrants are from the continent of Africa. Thirty-five percent are from the Pacific region. At least 77 languages are spoken in homes across Louisville. To improve its quality measures and deliver care in this environment, Norton Healthcare will need to conform to the CLAS.

## INTEGRATING MENTAL HEALTH AND MEDICAL SERVICES

The process of developing locally acceptable approaches to disparities requires dedicated organizations and financial resources. The Foundation for a Healthy Kentucky is an example of such an organization. Along with the efforts of Foundation for a Healthy Kentucky, Shelia Schuster is a leading advocate in this community for mental illness care. In Kentucky, as in many communities, public and private insurance plans treat coverage of mental illness care differently than it does chronic disease. For example, a person with a diagnosis of manic depressive illness is usually limited to 20 visits per year. The copayment for each office visit for treatment is 50 percent. If the person had diabetes, there would be no limit on the number of office visits. Most employer-sponsored health plans have a copayment for an office visit related to diabetes of 15 to 20 percent. Furthermore, persons with a diagnosis of a mental illness cannot receive treatment during a single visit for any accompanying medical illnesses. If you have a diagnosis of both manic depressive disease and diabetes, you cannot be treated for problems related to both during the same visit. This makes controlling each of these chronic diseases problematic. The limitations surrounding access to integrated care for the mentally ill have been a focal point for her advocacy. Her work spans years. Foundation for a Healthy Kentucky is an outgrowth of her work. It was established in 2001 with funds from the settlement agreement between the Commonwealth of Kentucky and Anthem, Inc. after Anthem's merger with Kentucky Blue Cross/Blue Shield. Its mission is to serve the unmet health care needs of Kentuckians. The Foundation for a Healthy Kentucky is concerned with *health policy, promoting lasting change in health care systems, improving access, reducing health disparities,* and *promoting health equity.* The Foundation for a Healthy Kentucky held a 2006 symposium, "No Wrong Door: Overcoming Obstacles to Integration of Mental Health and Medical Services." This symposium explored ways to remove the regulatory and reimbursement barriers that block service integration for persons with mental illness and accompanying medical problems. In 2010, the Foundation for a Healthy Kentucky convened public forum entitled Commonwealth Common Health. Susan Zepeda is the current president and CEO of this community-based organization. The commentaries from this meeting are being studied by health care delivery systems across the state. Does the ACA contain provisions that will support their efforts? Yes.

During the period between 2008 and 2011, two pieces of federal legislation were passed that created parity between mental health insurance coverage and physical health insurance coverage. The Wellstone Domenici Mental Health Parity and Addiction Equity Act of 2008 (Public Law 110-343 122 Stat. 3765) was passed in the fall of 2008. This act targets large employer insurance plans and Medicaid-managed care plans. It became effective on October 3, 2009. The ACA completed the removal of this barrier to mental health care by including mental health and substance care in Title I (Section 1302—Essential Benefits).

## SUMMARY

The quality movement in U.S. health care is a newly evolving effort that dates back to the 1990s. The quality movement would not have been possible if medical research had not made a commitment to the ethical conduct of research on human subjects. This was an important transition and the result of health care professionals acknowledging their role in inequity. Henry Beecher came to understand that his own behavior in the conduct of anesthesia research did not respect the rights and dignity of his patients. As a result, we now have a global commitment to safety, beneficence, and justice in medical research. Health care inequity is not a different issue from the ethical conduct of medical research. We are at the beginning of a process of quality in the delivery of health care. The issues surrounding health literacy and language-appropriate care are within the responsibility of providers to address. Currently, there is resistance to the implementation of CLAS. As health care delivery systems develop processes to minimize this barrier, providers will begin to use the process. They will come to understand—just as researchers have—that communication is central to quality care. Furthermore, it is not enough to say that the groups of individuals have poor outcomes because they are illiterate or undereducated. Communication is the primary responsibility of the provider. If a person is deaf, shouting will not work. If a person is blind, written pamphlets will not work. The process of communication permeates every aspect of health care. In a society as pluralistic as the United States, a commitment to communication is hard work. After all, Louisville, Kentucky, has 77 different languages spoken in homes across the county. It is not a coastal town. Its history does not include the experience with immigrants that larger cities like New York and San Francisco have. It will take time, financing, and a commitment to quality to overcome the local communication barriers. Eventually, health care delivery systems like Norton will need to engage native speakers from each of these language communities to develop solutions that increase patient satisfaction with care. This engagement will be reflected in their CAHPS scores. Norton physician practice improvements for these communities will be reflected in their Healthcare Effectiveness Data and Information Set scores.

The National Healthcare Quality Report shows that some Americans have difficulty accessing care. Once inside a health care organization, sometimes the treatment a patient receives is not appropriate. It is delivered in a language that cannot be understood by the patient. Title III of the ACA is dedicated to statutes defining quality health care in public plans. In the United States, facilities that receive public funds also treat patients with private insurance. Quality, then, becomes broadly disseminated throughout health care. Quality has the potential to diminish the health care inequities underlying disparity. With transparent reporting practices and measurement of patient satisfaction, in time we will know if this promise is achieved.

## BIBLIOGRAPHY

Agency for Healthcare Research and Quality (AHRQ). "2009 National Healthcare Quality & Disparities Reports." U.S. Department of Health and Human Services, 2010.

Agency for Healthcare Research and Quality (AHRQ). "Consumer Assessment Health Providers and Systems (CAHPS) Surveys and Tools to Advance Patient-Centered Care," https://www.cahps.ahrq.gov/default.asp.

American College of Physicians. "Screening for Prostate Cancer," http://www.acponline.org.

American Medical Association. "Prescription for a Healthier Practice: Physician Claims Process Check-Up," edited by claims checklist, 2008.

Beecher, Henry K. "Ethics and Clinical Research." *New England J Medicine* 274, no. 24 (1966): 1354–60.

Bennett, Paul G. "VA Health Economics Bulletin: Guidebook for Research Use of Paid Data," Health Economics Resource Center, 2, Menlo Park, 2009.

Boukus, Ellyn, and Peter J. Cunningham. "Mixed Signals: Trends in Americans' Access to Medical Care, 2007–2010." *Health Systems Change: Community Tracking Study Household Survey.* Tracking Report No. 25, 2011, http://www.hschange.com/CONTENT/1233.

Byrd, W. Michael, and Linda A. Clayton. *An American Health Dilemma: Race, Medicine, and Health Care in the United States 1900–2000.* New York: Routledge, 2002.

Campbell, Paul Erwin, Eugene C. Fitzhugh, Kathleen C. Brown, Shannon Looney, and Timothy Forde. "Health Disparities in Rural Areas: The Interaction of Race, Socioeconomic Status, and Geography." *Journal of Health Care for the Poor and Underserved* 21 (2010): 931–45.

Castillo, Lesley S., Brie A. Williams, Sarah M. Hooper, Charles P. Sabatino, Lois A. Weithorn, and Rebecca L. Sudore. "Lost in Translation: The Unintended Consequences of Advance Directive Law on Clinical Care." *Annals of Internal Medicine* 154, no. 2 (2011): 121–28.

Centers for Medicare & Medicaid Services. "Medicare Program; Clarifying Policies Related to the Responsibilities of Medicare-Participating Hospitals in

Treating Individuals with Emergency Medical Conditions." *CMS-1063-F,* Centers for Medicare & Medicaid Services, 162, Federal Register, 2011.

Centers for Medicare & Medicaid Services. "Medicare Program; Medicare Shared Savings Program: Accountable Care Organizations." *42 CFR Part 425,* Department of Health and Human Services, 127, Federal Register, 2011.

Centers for Medicare & Medicaid Services. "Premier Hospital Historical Data." U.S. Department of Health & Human Services, https://www.cms.gov/HospitalQualityInits/40_HospitalPremierHistoricalData.asp.

Cossman, J. S., W. L. James, A. G. Cosby, and R. E. Cossman. "Underlying Causes of the Emerging Nonmetropolitan Mortality Penalty." *Am J Public Health* 100, no. 8 (2010): 1417–19.

Dailey, Barbara. "Quality Measurement and Improvement in Medicaid and Chip: A New Journey," Evaluation Division of Quality, and Health Outcomes, Family and Children's Health Programs Group, Center for Medicaid, CHIP & Survey & Certification, Centers for Medicare & Medicaid Services, 2010.

Diamond, L. C., A. Wilson-Stronks, and E. A. Jacobs. "Do Hospitals Measure up to National Culturally and Linguistically Appropriate Service Standards?" *Medical Care* 48, no. 12 (2010): 8.

Eszter, Hargittai. "Second Level Digital Divide: Differences in People's Online Skills." *First Monday* (2002), http://www.citeulike.org/user/pajoma/article/3501930.

Fisher, Elliott S., David C. Goodman, and Amitabh Chandra. "Regional and Racial Variation in Health Care among Medicare Beneficiaries: A Brief Report of the Dartmouth Atlas Project." In *Aligning Forces for Quality: Improving Health and Health Care in Communities across America,* edited by Kristen K. Bronner. Princeton, NJ: Robert Wood Johnson Foundation, 2008.

Foundation for a Healthy Kentucky. "The Health of Kentucky: A County Assessment." Kentucky Institute of Medicine, 2007.

Foundation for a Healthy Kentucky. "Commonwealth, Common Health: Kentucky Conversations for Health Action." *Issue,* 2010.

Frei, C. R., E. M. Mortensen, L. A. Copeland, R. T. Attridge, M. J. Pugh, M. I. Restrepo, A. Anzueto, B. Nakashima, and M. J. Fine. "Disparities of Care for African Americans and Caucasians with Community Acquired Pneumonia: A Retrospective Cohort Study." *BMC Health Services Research* 10 (2010): 143.

Galvin, Robert S., and Elizabeth A. McGlynn. "Using Performance Measurement to Drive Improvement: A Road Map for Change." *Medical Care* 41, no. 1 (2003): I48–I60.

Ghazal, Maria. "Rin 0938-Aq17 Comments Re: Proposed Rule for Medicare Program; Availability of Medicare Data for Performance Measurement, 76 Fed. Reg. 33566 (June 8, 2011)." Department of Health and Human Services Centers for Medicare and Medicaid Services, *Business Roundtable* (2011): 5. Published electronically August 3, 2011, http://businessroundtable.org/news-center/business-roundtable-letter-on-proposed-rule-for-medicare-program/.

Greenberg, Greg A., Robert A. Rosenheck, Martin Peter Charns. "From Profession-Based Leadership to Service Line Management in the Veterans Health Administration: Impact on Mental Health Care." *Medical Care* 41, no. 9 (2003): 1013–23.

Hall M. J., C. J. DeFrances, S. N. Williams, A. Golosinskiy, and A. Schwartzman. "National Hospital Discharge Survey: 2007 Summary." National Center for Health Statistics, 21, 2010.

Hynes, Denise M., Duane Cowper, Michael Kerr, Joseph Kubal, and Patricia A. Murphy. "Database and Informatics Support Queri: Current Systems and Future Needs." *Medical Care* 38, no. QUERI Supplement I114–I128 (2000).

Jack, Brian W., Veerappa K. Chetty, David Anthony, Jeffrey L. Greenwald, Gail M. Sanchez, Anna E. Johson, Shaula R. Forsythe, Julie K. O'Donnell, Michael K. Paasche-Orlow, Christopher Manasseh, Stephen Martin, and Larry Culpepper. "A Reengineered Hospital Discharge Program to Decrease Rehospitalization. Clinical Trials Registration Number: Nct00252057." *Annals of Internal Medicine* 150 (2009): 178–87.

Johnson, Randel K., and Katie Mahoney. "Re: Proposed Rule Regarding the Availability of Medicare Data for Performance Measurement." U.S. Chamber of Commerce, 2011, http://www.uschamber.com.

Joynt K. E., E. J. Orav, and A. Jha. "Thirty-Day Readmission Rates for Medicare Beneficiaries by Race and Site of Care." *Journal of American Medical Association* 305, no. 7 (2011): 675–81.

Kressin, Nancy R., Urlike Boehmer, Dan Berlowitz, Cindy L. Christiansen, Arkadiy Pittman, and Judith A. Jones. "Racial Variations in Dental Procedures: The Case of Root Canal Therapy Versus Tooth Extraction." *Medical Care* 41, no. 11 (2003): 1256–61.

Kutner, Mark, Elizabeth Greenberg, Ying Jin, and Christine Paulsen. "The Health Literacy of America's Adults: Results from the 2003 National Assessment of Adult Literacy." U.S. Department of Education: National Center for Educational Statistics, Institute of Education Sciences, 2006.

Levinson, Daniel R. *Adverse Events in Hospitals: National Incidence among Medicare Beneficiaries.* OEI-06-09-00090. Washington, DC: Office of the Inspector General, 2010.

Lichtenberg, Frank R. "The Quality of Medical Care, Behavioral Risk Factors, and Longevity Growth." *International Journal of Health Care Finance and Economics* 11 (2011): 1–34.

McDonough, John E., Brian K. Gibbs, Janet L. Scott-Harris, Amanda M. Navarro, Karl Kronebusch, and Kimá Taylor. "A State Policy Agenda to Eliminate Racial and Ethnic Health Disparities." The Commonwealth Fund, 83, 2004.

McGlynn, Elizabeth A. "The Case for Keeping Quality on the Health Reform Agenda. Testimony Presented before the Senate Committee on Finance." RAND, 2008.

MEDPAC. "Data Book: Healthcare Spending and the Medicare Program. Chapter 4." MEDPAC, 12, 2010.

Mehrotra, A., M.C. Wang, J.R. Lave, J.L. Adams, and E.A. McGlynn. "Retail Clinics, Primary Care Physicians, and Emergency Departments: A Comparison of Patients' Visits." *Health Affairs (Millwood)* 27, no. 5 (2008): 1272–82.

Merrill C.T., P.L. Owens, and C. Stocks. "Emergency Department Visits for Adults in Community Hospitals from Selected States, 2005. HCUP Statistical Brief #47," 12, Agency for Healthcare Research and Quality, Rockville, MD, 2008.

Miles, Toni P., and Karla Washington. "Physical Problems Shaping Transitions of Care." In *Annual Review of Gerontology and Geriatrics,* edited by Peggye Dilworth-Anderson. New York, NY: Springer, 2011 (Chapter 4).

National Committee for Quality Assurance. "Health Plan Report Card," http://reportcard.ncqa.org/plan/external/.

Nicholas, Lauren H., Kenneth M. Langa, Theodoe J. Iwashyna, and David R. Weir. "Regional Variation in the Association between Advance Directives and End-of-Life Medicare Expenditures." *Journal of the American Medical Association* 306, no. 13 (2011): 1447–53.

Niederdeppe, Jeff Q., Lisa Bu, Porismita Borah, David A. Kindig, and Stephanie A. Robert. "Message Design Strategies to Raise Public Awareness of Social Determinants of Health and Population Health Disparities." *The Millbank Quarterly* 86, no. 3 (2008): 481–513.

NTOCC Performance & Metrics Work Group. "Improving on Transitions of Care: How to Implement and Evaluate a Plan," 2008.

O'Connell, Joan, Yi Rong, Charlton Wilson, Spero Munson, and Kelly J. Acton. "Racial Disparities in Health Status: A Comparison of the Morbidity among American Indians and United States Adults with Diabetes." *Diabetes Care* 33 (2010): 1463–70.

Office of Minority Health. "National Standards for Culturally and Linguistically Appropriate Services in Health Care," 2001.

Office of Minority Health. "National Study of Culturally and Linguistically Appropriate Services in Managed Care Organization (CLAS in MCOs Study)," 2003.

Petersen, Laura A., Steven M Wright, Eric D Peterson, and Jennifer Daley. "Impact of Race on Cardiac Care and Outcome in Veterans with Acute Myocardial Infarction." *Medical Care* 40, Suppl. 1 (2002): I86–I96. Published electronically January 2002.

Pries J.L., C. Cook, S.P. Burch, and C.R. Cantrell. "Racial Differences in Quality Care Measures, Medication Adherence, Health Care Costs, and Utilization with Common Chronic Diseases in a 9-State Medicaid Population." Paper presented at the American Public Health Association 137th Annual Meetings, Philadelphia, 2009.

Rebhun, Uzi, and Adi Raveh. "The Spatial Distribution of Quality of Life in the United States and Interstate Migration, 1965–1970 and 1985–1990." *Social Indicators Research* 78, no. 1 (2006): 137–78.

Rollow, W., T.R. Lied, P. McGann, et al. "Assessment of the Medicare Quality Improvement Organization Program." *Annals of Internal Medicine* 145 (2006): 12.

Schoenberg, N.E., S.H. Bardach, K.N. Manchikanti, and A.C. Goodenow. "Appalachian Residents' Experiences with and Management of Multiple Morbidity." *Qualitative Health Research* 21, no. 5 (May 2011): 601–11.

Shih, Anthony, Karen Davis, Stephen C. Schoenbaum, Anne Gauthier, Rachel Nuzum, and Douglas McCarthy. "Organizing the United States Health Care Delivery System for High Performance," edited by Martha Hostetter, The Commonwealth Fund, Washington, DC, 2008.

Shin, Hyron, and Robert A. Kominski. "Language Use in the United States: 2007." American Community Survey Reports, 2010.

Simonds, Vanessa W., Graham A. Colditz, Rima E. Rudd, and Thomas D. Sequist. "Cancer Screening among Native Americans in California." *Ethnicity & Disease* 21, no. 2 (2011): 202–09.

Slack, C.W., and W.V. Slack. "The United Countries of America: Benchmarking the Quality of US Health Care." *Mayo Clinic Proceedings* 86, no. 8 (2011): 788–90.

Smith, Alexander K., Rebecca L. Sudore, and Eliseo J. Perez-Stable. "Palliative Care for Latino Patients and Their Families: 'Whenever We Prayed, She Wept.'" *Journal of the American Medical Association* 301, no. 10 (2009): 1047–E1.

Sullivan, E., S. Braithwaite, K. Dietz, and C. Hickey. "Health Services Utilization and Medical Costs among Medicare Atrial Fibrillation Patients." *AF Stat*: Avalere Health LLC Supported by Sanofi-Adventis, United States LLC., 2010.

Title 45 Cfr Part Code of Federal Regulations: Title 45 Public Welfare Department of Health and Human Services Part 46 Protection of Human Subjects. Effective July 14, 2009.

U.S. Department of Commerce. "Falling through the Net: Defining the Digital Divide," 1999, http://www.ntia.doc.gov/legacy/ntiahome/fttn99/contents.html.

U.S. Department of Health and Human Services. "Indian Health Care Improvement Act Made Permanent." Health and Human Services, http://www.hhs.gov/news/press/2010pres/03/20100326a.html.

Vaughn, Thomas E., Kimberly D. McCoy, Bonnie J. BootsMiller, Robert F. Woolson, Bernard Sorofman, Toni Tripp-Reimer, Jonathan Perlin, and Bradley N.

Doebbeling. "Organizational Predictors of Adherence to Ambulatory Care Screening Guidelines." *Medical Care* 40, no. 40 (2002): 1172–85.

Wailoo, Keith. *Dying in the City of the Blues: Sickle Cell Anemia and the Politics of Race and Health*. Chapel Hill, NC: The University of North Carolina Press, 2001.

Wennberg, John E., Annette M. O'Connor, E. Dale Collins, and James N. Weinstein. "Extending the P4P Agenda, Part 1: How Medicare Can Improve Patient Decision Making and Reduce Unnecessary Care." *Health Affairs* 26, no. 6 (2007): 1564–674, http://content.healthaffairs.org/content/26/6/1564.full.

Wennberg, John E., Elliott S. Fisher, Jonathan S. Skinner, and Kristen K. Bronner. "Extending the P4P Agenda, Part 2: How Medicare Can Reduce Waste and Improve the Care of the Chronically Ill." *Health Affairs* 26, no. 6 (2007): 1575–85, http://content.healthaffairs.org/content/26/6/1575.abstract.

White, S., and Dillow, S. "Key Concepts and Features of the 2003 National Assessment of Adult Literacy (NCES 2006-471)." U.S. Department of Education. Washington, DC. National Center for Education Statistics, 2005.

# CHAPTER 4

## Business Models, Disparity, and Reform

Health disparities are a public health problem. Their resolution requires a population level approach. In this chapter, we review the business operations of public hospitals, public health plans, and private businesses that occupy a niche market of service to the poor. There is evidence to suggest that individual public hospitals are too small to operate effectively in a health care delivery market dominated by chronic disease. Are there successful business plans that are also dedicated to public health? Market size is at the heart of any thoughtful business plan. Estimating the size of U.S. health disparities makes creating a business plan to serve this market difficult. It includes 47 million uninsured persons. The underinsured persons with incomplete health insurance benefits number 70 to 80 million. There are also illegal immigrants who access our health care delivery system. These numbers are too big for a business plan with a focus on a single hospital and its satellite clinics. Unfortunately, our public conversation about health care access is based on stories about single hospital closures:

> A safety net hospital falls into financial crisis.
> Shaila Dewan and Kevin Sack, *New York Times,*
> January 8, 2008

> Will safety net hospitals survive health reform? Experts worry expanding insurance coverage will force such centers to close.
> *Associated Press,* msnbc, September 8, 2009

Catholic Health Partners looks to sell Pennsylvania group.
*Business Journals,* October 11, 2010

Hospital closings jeopardize care in ethnic communities.
America's Wire/New America Media,
Marjorie Valburn, January 20, 2011

The individual institutions covered in these stories are familiar to their communities. Each hospital occupies an important place in the history of U.S. health care. After the Hill–Burton Construction Act of 1946, the public hospital model for health care delivery to the poor expanded to occupy many large cities in the United States. These institutions were found in places like Atlanta, Miami, Memphis, Chicago, Los Angeles, and New Orleans. With each subsequent turn in the 50-year history of health care reform, there is debate about the need for their continued existence. After the enactment of Medicaid and Medicare in 1964, a number of these hospitals closed. The hospital formerly known as Martin Luther King Jr./Drew Medical Center in South Los Angeles closed in 2007. The Joint Commission on Hospital Accreditation refused to renew its license to operate due to violations of patient care standards. There are plans to reopen the facility in 2013. Within the context of this discussion, it could be said that their model of operation lacked sufficient financing. Public hospitals have always focused on crisis-driven care. These institutions were conceived during an historical period when crises were composed of infectious disease outbreaks or mass immigrations. During the 1940s, almost 60 percent of the U.S. population was under the age of 35. In 1940, the average life expectancy from birth was almost 63 years of age—61 years for men and 65 years for women. In 2010, the average life expectancy in the United States was 78 years of age. In 1940, women were more likely to die in childbirth—317 per 100,000. Today, that figure is 13 per 100,000. Since the development of public hospitals, the pattern of disease in the United States has evolved from one dominated by infectious diseases to one dominated by chronic conditions. Over the 50-year period, our public hospitals have struggled to adapt to these changing disease patterns. Public hospitals do not have the funds to update their infrastructure when needed.

What about the business model of public hospitals? The net revenues for the National Association of Public Hospitals and Health Systems (NAPH) members amounted to 40 billion dollars in 2008, an average of 454 million dollars each. These hospitals continue to rely on a combination of federal, state, and local funds to sustain their operations. In 2008, the revenue stream consisted of Medicaid (33%), Medicare (21%), and state or local payments (13%). An additional 26 percent of revenues came from commercially insured patients. Payments from uninsured patients—self pay— accounted for 4 percent of net revenues. There is considerable variation in size among NAPH members. The largest public hospitals in the United States have revenue of more than one billion dollars (2008). These institutions include Jackson Memorial Hospital in Miami, Florida (1.5 billion dollars); The Ohio State University Medical Center (1.3 billion dollars); University of Massachusetts Medical Center (1.2 billion dollars); Los Angeles County and University of Southern California Medical Center (1.1 billion dollars); and Boston Medical Center (one billion dollars). The Harris County Hospital District (Houston, Texas) reported slightly more than 900 million dollars. The remaining public hospitals reported revenues of less than 900 million dollars. Are the individual public hospitals too small to operate effectively in a health care delivery market dominated by chronic disease? What does a self-sustaining delivery system look like? Can anyone operate a delivery system to care for the nation's most complex patients?

Financing for each public hospital includes government supplemental payments known as disproportionate share hospital (DSH). The disproportionate share hospital payment portion of the Omnibus Budget Reconciliation Act of 1981 recognized the need to take into account the hospitals serving a disproportionate number of low-income patients with special needs. Safety net hospitals, as public hospitals are now called, continue to serve as a gateway to health care. Many are located in urban neighborhoods. Some of these institutions are required to accept all patients. Others are privately owned hospitals that disproportionately serve the uninsured. One concern shared by the CEOs of public hospitals is the way the ACA treats disproportionate share hospital payments. Over an extended period, the ACA reduces disproportionate share hospital payment (Sections 1203 and 2551). The logic underlying this policy is simple. Expanding health insurance should reduce the need for disproportionate share hospital payment support. CEOs of public hospitals refer to the experience of public hospitals in Massachusetts during the state's health care reform. There is consensus that the ACA will not eliminate the need for disproportionate share hospital payment because it does not completely resolve the role that public hospitals play. These hospitals are one part of the U.S. health care system. Disproportionate share hospital payment is one policy in 2,400 pages of law. Disproportionate share hospital payment only addresses the needs of the 13,000 or more member institutions of the National Association of Public Hospitals. Disproportionate share hospital payment policy aims at a small piece of health care inequity and is only a Band-Aid for the larger problem of health care inequity.

This chapter moves beyond that debate. Are there business models that focus on the modern pattern of illness among the uninsured, underinsured, and illegal immigrants? The answer to this question is "Yes." Like all health care businesses, these companies are either insurance companies or health care delivery systems. One common characteristic of these businesses is their multiple state operations. These are niche market companies. Their structure resembles traditional businesses with a product of insurance or health care delivery. Insurance companies collect premiums and negotiate with vendors to provide the goods and services used in health care. The delivery system takes care of everything else. BlueCross BlueShield, United Healthcare, Aetna are all insurance companies. Geisinger Health System, Intermountain Healthcare, Mayo Clinics are examples of delivery systems. This chapter takes a detailed look at the financing and structure of companies that make a commitment to care for the poor.

## MEDICAID-MANAGED CARE COMPANIES

Let us start with business models for health insurance. The health insurance business model has a simple financing and profit-generation structure. A traditional insurance company receives funds from two sources: investors and member premiums. The investors expect a profit. The group paying premiums expects to have health care. The pooled funds pay for the goods and services used by members of the group. The remaining funds go to investors as profit. Profits can be improved by increasing premiums, controlling the payout for health care, or enrolling more individuals in the plan. Balancing the satisfaction of insurance customers and investors is critical to a successful health insurance business. In the United States, almost 77 percent of adults obtain their health insurance through their employers. Health insurance customers in the U.S. markets include both employees and employers. Premium increases either cover the cost of health care or support investor earnings. Prior to the ACA, there was no limit to profit-taking from pooled premiums. Section 2718 of the ACA requires that private plans allocate at least 85 percent of premium funds toward member health care costs—*medical loss ratio*. A medical loss ratio favoring consumers immediately increases the funds available to pay for care. This section of the ACA could potentially improve the satisfaction of insurance customers with their plans. The ACA has the potential to expand private plan enrollments. Insurance companies can no longer use preexisting medical conditions to deny coverage. Although there are arguments about additional costs associated with these customers, the additional enrollees could increase investor profits.

There are private companies that specialize in managed Medicaid insurance plans. These are niche market companies. Their niche is developing health insurance for local and state government programs. Just like other private health insurance companies, they worry about balancing finance and profit generation. Unlike the other ones, these companies operate within the tight fiscal boundaries of government finances. Their ability to increase premiums is limited. To successfully negotiate health care for members of public plans, these companies need business plans that accommodate fluctuations in their financing stream that consists of taxes and premiums. Yes, enrollees in both Medicare and Medicaid pay health insurance premiums. The ACA contains provisions to provide federal subsidies for the premium payments of low-wage workers up to 400 percent of the federal poverty level. There are also limits to the types of strategies that a business could use to reduce health care costs. The contracts developed by managed Medicaid companies cannot be longer than two years. Most states have biennial budget cycles. Many states have constitutions that do not allow for deficit spending. There is always the possibility that a state could renegotiate its contract in the middle of a budget cycle. Before the ACA, states routinely balanced their Medicaid budgets by changing income eligibility criteria for enrollees. For example, a state sets income eligibility at 185 percent of the federal poverty level. That works out to 33,000 for a family of three. The next year it might be decreased to 133 percent of the federal poverty level to meet a budget shortfall. To the individual, this shift means that one year you are on Medicaid, the next year you are not. To obtain matching federal funds, state Medicaid programs must supply coverage to mandatory populations—children, pregnant women, the disabled, the aged, and the blind. Before the ACA, childless adults were designed *optional* populations. When state funding was available, this group might receive Medicaid coverage. When state funds were tight—like they are now—this group was denied Medicaid coverage. In 2014, Medicaid will undergo fundamental changes to establish national eligibility levels and add covered benefits. In return, states will receive increased matching federal funds for the cost of covering childless adults and many parents of children. The additional funds for these initiatives will be drawn from reduced hospital disproportionate share payments and other regulations designed to improve the stability of Medicaid-managed care plans. There is one more concern. During the period before expansion, states and their managed Medicaid contractors are faced with a prohibition that blocks states from cutting Medicaid eligibility. This policy has been termed *maintenance of effort*. In the period before 2014, the only avenues open to the states and their managed Medicaid contractors are reducing provider reimbursement rates and reducing or eliminating covered benefits. All of these issues—state budgets, federal supplements, and required populations—create a landscape that is discouraging for most traditional profit-driven businesses. Therefore, why would anyone get into the managed Medicaid business?

Behind every business are leaders with a philosophy. Get their stories, and the rationale for their involvement in a type of business becomes a little clearer. In the current health care environment, many physicians, hospitals, and other businesses are publically refusing to treat uninsured, underinsured, and illegal immigrant populations. It is legitimate to ask, "Who would lead a company with this clientele as its core business?" There are three large-scale competitors in the managed Medicaid care marketplace—Centene Corporation, Molina Healthcare, and AmeriHealth Mercy.

Centene Corporation is based in St. Louis, Missouri, and has 4,200 employees. Its CEO, Michael Neidorff, has been at the helm of Centene since 2005. In 2010, Centene provided Medicaid coverage for almost two million persons. Texas and Georgia are its biggest markets and account for 48 percent of the total members served by Centene health plans. This is what he says about Centene:

> I'm very proud that we have an organization committed to helping insure that the disadvantaged receive the highest quality care.

Its corporate website describes its mission using a similar language:

> [We] will provide better health at lower costs. Centene works with states to create solutions . . . that address the distinct needs of [Medicaid and uninsured] populations.

In 2010, Centene reported sales of almost four and a half billion dollars and a *one-year sales growth* of 8 percent. Whether you measure profit as *net income* (more than 94 million dollars), *one-year net income growth*

(13%), *return on invested capital* (7.5%), or *net profit margin* (2%), 2010 was a good year for Centene.

Another corporation in the Medicaid-managed care business is Molina Healthcare. The president and CEO is Joseph Mario Molina. He is the son of founder C. David Molina. Dr. Molina is a trained endocrinologist and has personal experience caring for patients. The Molina website lists his numerous awards. In 2005, *Time* magazine listed him as one of the 25 most influential Hispanics in America. When discussing his core business, he sounds like any other CEO. The following is text from a transcript of the 2010 second quarter earnings conference call:

> [We saw] a forty percent improvement over the second quarter of 2010. We are pleased with these results, which reflect our continued strength and momentum in the Medicaid space. . . . Even more exciting are the many opportunities over the next few years. These include upcoming Medicaid managed care procurements, A[ged], B[lind], D[isabled] population expansions, dual eligible special needs plans expansions, and the Medicaid Management Information System procurements.

Clearly, Dr. Molina does not view Medicaid enrollees as a drag on the health care system. The Molina Healthcare website echoes his enthusiasm:

> [We are] a multistate healthcare organization with flexible care delivery systems focused exclusively on government sponsored healthcare programs for low income families and individuals.

What was 2010 like for Molina Healthcare? In a word, 2010 was profitable. The health plan covered 1.6 million members. Their reported sales were 4 billion dollars with a net income of 55 million, a net profit margin of 1.5 percent, and a return on invested capital of 7.5 percent. Molina Healthcare employs approximately 4,000 persons, and its members live mostly in the states of Washington, California, and Ohio.

The third company is AmeriHealth Mercy. In 2009, Michael Rashid was named its CEO. Prior to becoming CEO, he served for 15 years as the company's executive vice president and chief operating officer. The only publically available source of financial data available for AmeriHealth Mercy is on the company's website. From its headquarters in Philadelphia, Pennsylvania, AmeriHealth Mercy has focused on Medicaid-managed care since 1983. It has more than 2,000 employees. The business serves four million Medicaid members through affiliated plans and products. These products go beyond insurance to include disease management and health outreach. Their website emphasizes this mission:

> We help people get care, stay well, and build healthy communities. We have a special concern for those who are poor.

This mission goes well beyond the core business of health insurance and into economic development. To understand that mission, consider the following commentary from Michael Rashid in a panel before the Congressional Black Caucus on September 23, 2011:

> Medicaid expenditures drive an important economic engine that supports hospitals, physicians, medical equipment providers, pharmacists, and nursing homes. In part, these expenditures have contributed to employment growth. . . . The [ACA] also provides for significant investments in community health centers, which have long been an important source of access to care for the nation's vulnerable populations. Over the next five years, the law provides eleven billion dollars in funding for the operation, expansion, and construction of community health centers nationally. These centers provide high quality jobs in many of the nation's most economically distressed communities.

He goes on to make the link between Medicaid and economic activity:

> In the communities where AmeriHealth Mercy is based, every Medicaid dollar spent generates almost three dollars more in economic activity . . . that in paying for member care, managed care organizations like AmeriHealth Mercy reinvest ninety three percent of the twelve billion dollars of federal Medicaid funding for Pennsylvania in local communities.

During his presentation, he makes this final point:

> Not only does Medicaid reduce health disparities, by virtue of those it serves, but it can also reduce economic disparities for women and minority owned business.

Each CEO—Neidorff, Molina, and Rashid—promotes a corporate model that recognizes the role of their business in the larger problem of health care access inequity. AmeriHealth Mercy, like Centene and Molina Health-care, serves millions of low-income Americans with a business model that keeps an eye on the bottom line.

## DELIVERY SYSTEMS

Health care delivery systems include the brick and mortar, personnel, and instruments of care. The large public hospitals *are* delivery systems. They provide hospital, outpatient, and community-based care. Jackson Memorial Hospital in Miami, Florida, is the largest public hospital in the United States. It was founded in 1918. In addition to payments from public and private insurances, it is supported by county residents through a sales tax of one-half cent. The hospital's finances are managed through the Public Health Trust of Miami Dade County. Jackson Memorial Hospital has 10,100 employees. According to Becker's Hospital Review, the system logged a surplus of four million dollars in June 2010. This surplus appeared after cleaning up its accounts receivable. Without the adjustment, the system would have lost 16 million dollars. How does this public hospital delivery system compare with private sector delivery systems whose core business is centered on a commitment to health care for the poor?

Catholic Health Partners is a private, not-for-profit organization with a stated commitment to care for the poor. Its headquarters are in Cincinnati, Ohio. Its facilities include 30 hospitals and more than a dozen long-term care facilities. It also operates affordable housing for the elderly and wellness centers. It employs almost 39,000 people across Ohio, Kentucky, and Tennessee. Sales during 2009 amounted to four billion dollars with a net profit margin of 9 percent. Michael Connelly is the CEO. During an interview, he commented on the issue of organization and size:

> size alone can't solve all problems . . . [but] the scale that an organization like Catholic Health Partners has is helpful in meeting the information technology and data sharing requirements of the new era in medicine.

Catholic Health Partners serves communities where health care reimbursements are lower than the national average—rural parts of northwestern and southwestern Ohio and eastern Kentucky. To run a stable system, sometimes there are tough choices:

> For more than two decades, hospitals [in the Scranton, Pennsylvania] area have endured lower than average reimbursements for care and

a static population base [due to an aging population]. This has, at times, resulted in empty hospital beds and the duplication of services.

In its 2010 report to the community, the CEO of Catholic Health Partners makes the following comment about the closure of Pennsylvania hospitals:

> In 2010, after prayerful consideration and exhausting all options, we announced our intention to sell our facilities in Northeast Pennsylvania and sell or enter into joint ventures for facilities in our Tennessee region. In both situations, we felt that we can best assure vibrant, healthy communities by stepping out of the way or partnering with organizations better positioned to create transformative change in these two communities. We anticipate that these transitions will occur in 2011. In both situations, our actions were driven by our commitment to improve the health of the communities we serve and to ensure the long-term viability of our mission.

Catholic Health Partners estimates that they provide one million dollars per day of free care and an additional community benefit of 365 million dollars to the areas they serve. This benefit is in the form of charity care and support for community programs. Gloria Bazzoli, a professor at Virginia Commonwealth University, has studied the closure of public hospitals in communities like Scranton, Pennsylvania. These closures increase the distance traveled for care by individuals most likely to have limited transportation—elderly and Medicaid enrollees. Is Catholic Health Partners too small to meet the needs of their core business?

Ascension Health is a private, not-for-profit health care delivery system. It is the largest Catholic hospital system in the United States. Its network consists of 70 general hospitals along with a dozen long-term care, acute care, rehabilitation, and psychiatric hospitals. It has a network of medical facilities that spans 20 states and the District of Columbia. The network is concentrated along the Mississippi Valley and western Ohio Valley with additional locations in Wisconsin, Michigan, Kansas, Texas, and the Northeast. This delivery system was created in 1999 from a union of the Daughters of Charity and the Sisters of St. Joseph. Anthony R. Tersigni was appointed CEO in 2004. Dr. Tersigni has a record of service in Catholic charitable organizations such as Society of St. Vincent de Paul, Catholic Health Association of the United States, The Catholic University of America, where he was a member of the Board of Trustees, and Legatus International, where he is a member of the Board of Governors. In its 2010 annual report, Ascension lists its total operating revenue at 15 billion dollars. Their website describes Ascension's mission as follows:

> Like other Catholic health care systems, Ascension is directed by the Church to care for those most in need. Our Catholic philosophy permeates our national health ministries and our promise to provide health care that works, health care that is safe, and health care that leaves no one behind.

In this report, Ascension estimates that more than one billion dollars was spent on care of the poor. Thirty-six percent of these funds went directly to the unpaid cost of public programs. Unlike Catholic Health Partners, there are no reports of facility sell-offs in the 12-month period between 2009 and 2010. Is Ascension large enough to sustain losses associated with uncompensated care without becoming unstable? Uncompensated care will always be a feature of U.S. delivery systems. Why was there not an open discussion about the business of providing uncompensated care during the ACA debate?

Kaiser Permanente is the only large-scale, private sector, nonchurch affiliated health care system in the United States with a mission statement that includes care for the poor. It combines health insurance with a health care delivery system. A not-for-profit business, it operates through a network of 36 hospitals, 600 medical offices, and 15,000 physicians. Its insurance plan covers almost nine million people. It was started in 1941 by Harold Hatch with a suggestion to Dr. Sidney Garfield. Dr. Garfield, so the story goes, was trying to keep his newly built Contractors General Hospital open for workers building the Los Angeles Aqueduct. He refused to turn away any sick or injured workers. Some of them did not have insurance, so he was left with no payment for his services. Harold Hatch, an engineer on the project, suggested that the insurance companies pay Dr. Garfield a fixed amount per day, per worker up front. This approach would solve the hospital's immediate money troubles and, at the same time, enable Dr. Garfield to emphasize maintaining health and safety rather than merely treating illness and injury. For five cents per day, workers were provided this new form of health coverage. For an additional five cents per day, workers could also receive coverage for any medical problems, not just the ones related to their jobs. Thousands of workers enrolled, and Dr. Garfield's hospital became a financial success. By 2009, the Kaiser Permanente Private Consortium made 42 billion dollars in sales and had a one-year sales growth of 4.5 percent.

Health and community service are the basis of Kaiser Permanente's core business. The largest concentration of plan participants is in Northern California—slightly more than three million persons or 40 percent of enrollees. To serve this population, the delivery system is organized into eight service areas with a Kaiser-affiliated medical center at its core. In addition to insurance and health care delivery, Kaiser conducts medical research and offers health education to the communities it serves. In 2009, the National Institutes of Health spent almost three billion dollars on research with a focus on health disparities. In the same year, Kaiser spent almost two billion dollars for community benefit, which included 124 million dollars for research, 81 million dollars for training programs of the health professionals, and 161 million dollars in grants and donations.

George Halvorson is the chairman and CEO of Kaiser Foundation Hospitals and Kaiser Foundation Health Plan, Inc. He has supervised the investment in electronic medical records, physician support systems, and quality improvement programs in the Kaiser system. Before joining Kaiser, he was part of the senior management staff at Blue Cross and Blue Shield of Minnesota. In 2009, he was interviewed by Ezra Klein of the *Washington Post* to discuss health insurance and integrated care. Health disparities are not a specific topic for discussion. He does, however, discuss public insurance plans, Medicare, and Medicaid.

**Ezra Klein (EK)**: Do we have a competitive insurance market in the United States?

**George Halvorson (GH)**: We need to do three things. Cover people. Fix care, focusing on the patients with chronic care, and set prices. But the thing is we have the highest prices in the world. The unit prices here are a multiple of any other country . . .

**EK**: . . . What people say is that you want a single payer system because you need, a large, central buyer to secure [low] prices . . .

**GH**: One of the reasons is that in the Netherlands, in Germany, the government sets the fee. In Canada, the government sets the fee. Each of those countries has said we'll have a single fee schedule.

**EK**: So when you say that we should have a public plan with Medicare rates, Karen Ignagni, who represents an organization [American Hospital Association] you're part of, says, "No, the only reason Medicare can pay so little is because we [private plans] pay so much." But doesn't Europe pay that much?

**GH**: All hospitals believe firmly that they lose money on Medicare and Medicaid. And I've run enough hospitals to know that's probably true. And there will be some cost shift. The other thing that's happening is we have the lowest hospital days in the world, but we have increased the rate of spending per day. . . . I recommend we do reduce the rate of increase for a number of years.

In part two of the interview, they discuss delivery system issues:

**EK**: Kaiser is one of the first major systems to convert entirely to electronic records. Why has that been so difficult?

**GH**: . . . I think like a minister of health. We have a population of more than eight million people in Kaiser, which is more than forty two states and one hundred countries, and we're an integrated care system. I'm always thinking in terms of population health. Within KP, when we started electronic medical records, some people wanted an oncology system and some wanted a surgery system, but putting it into separate pieces would have been wrong.

**EK**: . . . Kaiser Permanente is an integrated care system. You have your own hospitals and doctors. It's not an insurer like Aetna is an insurer.

**GH**: We are a single payer system unto ourselves. For us, a hospital or an imaging center is a cost center, not a profit center. We'll have one clinic shared by a hospital and a couple of specialties, while in the fee for service world, each of the specialties might have their own CT scanners so they can bill off them. We have a lot of CT scanners, too. We probably do more of them than any other private organization in the world. But, we do them for the patients, so the CT information is shared and they don't need to be repeated. That makes us different than folks who want to deliver great care but are organized around billing systems. . .

**EK**: A number of the organizations that are considered the best and most cost efficient in the United States—Kaiser, Mayo, the Veterans Health Administration—are integrated at a level that's really quite rare. Normally, you'd expect that to give them a competitive advantage and they'd eventually take over the market. But that doesn't seem to happen. Why?

**GH**: Well, the VA has its own population. When you look at the Mayos of the world, they're doing well. They have a good business model that's working for them. But everyone else has a good business model that's working for them, too. There are two and a half trillion dollars in this market. There's no reason, if you have a comfortable cash flow, why would you do hard things and heavy lifting to get to a different model?

Avoiding the costs associated with uncompensated care is a concern for private insurance plans and delivery systems. For George Halvorson and Kaiser, uncompensated care is a population problem. Population problems are approached with community-based interventions. The Kaiser business model includes investments outside of the hospital frame of reference. With an integrated system of insurance and delivery, Kaiser Permanente appears to be large enough to take on the work of resolving the uncompensated health care problem of the United States.

The Veterans Health Administration (VHA) is the highest-rated health care system in the United States. Its size and structure more closely resemble Kaiser Permanente. The VHA includes more than 1,400 hospitals, clinics, and nursing homes; 14,800 doctors; 61,000 nurses, and more than 6 million patients. Robert A. Petzel is the current VHA undersecretary for health. He occupies a cabinet-level position. Being a member of the president's cabinet adds political pressure to existing health care delivery issues. VHA patients are mostly male and embody many of the characteristics that make health disparity population complex—homelessness, disability, drug abuse, psychiatric illness, and chronic disease. These veterans also have complex mental and physical injuries obtained during their military service. The VHA has the largest geriatric population base in the country. The average age of the World War II veteran is 82 years. The Vietnam-era veterans are part of the baby boom cohort and are entering an age where chronic disease increases. There are new challenges for the VHA from veterans returning from Afghanistan and Iraq with disability caused by head injuries that would have killed a person in previous wars. Despite all of these challenges, patient ratings in the VHA are the highest for any health care system in the United States. What can public hospitals learn from the VHA?

The VHA was organized into 22 regional networks called Veterans Integrated Service Networks (VISNs) in 1995. Most VISNs consist of 7 to 10 hospitals, 25 to 30 ambulatory care clinics, 4 to 7 nursing homes, and 1 to 2 affordable housing units. The number of VHA hospitals was cut in half between 1995 and 2010 as its model of care shifted toward prevention. The key to reduction in service and improvement in patient satisfaction is the VHA's quality improvement initiative. This initiative is designed to recognize outstanding performance in the health care workforce with financial rewards. The maximum awards for one program are

25,000 dollars per facility and 5,000 dollars per person. The VHA encourages competition between VISNs as well as a general competition for the best metrics. The U.S. Department of Veterans Affairs operates a system of 153 medical centers, 882 ambulatory care and community based outpatient clinics, 207 centers for veterans, 136 nursing homes, 45 residential rehabilitation treatment programs, and 92 comprehensive home-based care programs—all providing medical and related services to eligible veterans. These facilities provide care in multiple settings—hospital, outpatient, laboratory, pharmacy, and custodial care. VHA facilities employ about 200,000 full-time equivalent employees. In 2006, there were approximately 24 million living veterans of the U.S. military. In that year, the department provided medical services to five million veterans and 400,000 other patients. There were an additional almost three million veterans enrolled in the system who did not seek service. During Hurricane Katrina in 2005, Gulf Coast veterans enrolled in the VHA and used the VHA electronic record system to maintain continuity of health care across the country.

In 1995 when the VHA began its quality improvement process, it also put into place measures of benefit. As the ambulatory care program began to ramp up, hospital-based care decreased. Between 1995 and 1998, there was a 62 percent decline in bed days of care per 1,000 patients and a parallel increase in ambulatory care visits of 43 percent. There were system-wide staffing reductions of 11 percent between 1994 and 1998. With the advent of electronic health records, more than 2,700 paperwork forms were eliminated. These changes are now embedded within the culture of VHA care. Studies in the medical literature provide evidence that significantly more patients receive recommended preventive, inpatient, and outpatient care at the VHA in 10 of 11 categories.

The Congressional Budget Office has estimated that the VHA's budget per enrollee grew by almost 2 percent from 1999 to 2005. This estimate is less than Medicare's rate of growth of 29 percent in cost per capita over that same period with a rate of more than 4 percent per year. One factor that has enabled the VHA to hold down its costs is the fact that federal law enables the department to purchase pharmaceutical products at the lowest prices of any U.S. delivery system. In addition, the VHA uses a restrictive formulary to reduce its pharmaceutical costs even further. In 2006, pharmaceuticals made up more than 13 percent of the VHA's medical expenditures, compared with 10 percent of total national health expenditures. The higher percentage for the department despite its lower acquisition costs may reflect its older population of patients. Some veterans rely on VHA for medications. They obtain health care elsewhere but get prescriptions at the VHA pharmacy because of its relatively low copayments.

## SUMMARY

Health disparities have always been a public health problem in the United States. The approach to resolving them has evolved as financing has become available. The public hospital model of health care dates back to the early 1900s. The finances of these institutions were unstable. Charity was the primary source of funds. Almost all the funds were used to purchase hands-on care because technology did not play a central role in health care. Medications were not a mainstay of care. Philanthropy was the only source of financing for medical research. See the discussion of the history of cancer research funding in chapter 5. In this early period, infections were the main cause of death at each stage of life. Infants died in the first year of life from whooping cough. Almost one-third of women died during childbirth. Young people died of influenza and pneumonia. The life expectancy in the United States was less than 50 years. Public health care systems were focused on supporting patients until the danger of immediate death was past. This meant keeping a person in the hospital and watching him or her closely. At the time, hospital-based care for the severely ill was new. The number of public hospitals increased once financing was stabilized with funds from Medicare and Medicaid. Once public financing stabilized health care delivery systems, infants were less likely to die. In a stable public care system, older adults without resources were able to get the hospital care they needed. In this same period, employer-sponsored insurance put more dollars into the health care system. These dollars fueled the growth of health care businesses. These businesses produce the durable goods and medicines routinely used in health care. Chronic diseases are now the dominating form of illness. There are disparities in the pattern of their distribution across the population. Unlike infectious disease, control of chronic conditions occurs over a prolonged period on the order of months to years. There are medications used to delay the onset of complications from these diseases. Chronic disease care drives total health care expenditures in the United States. The U.S. public health care delivery system retains much of its historical structure of hospital-based, emergency-focused care. Public hospitals are having a difficult time adapting to the needs of chronic disease care.

If you have high blood pressure, diabetes, or arthritis, you have a chronic disease. If you take medication on a daily basis for any condition, you are receiving chronic medical care. Asthma and chronic obstructive pulmonary disease—sometimes called COPD—are chronic diseases. Symptoms like joint or back pain that you experience on a regular basis are a type of chronic disease. If you are consistently having difficulty sleeping, you have a chronic disease. All of these conditions as well as unnamed others are successfully managed with coordinated medical care. Success is measured by minimizing the impact of illness. Persons with successful chronic disease management are able to lead active lives. They are able to care for their children, perform in the workplace, and contribute their time and talents to their communities. Chronic disease management is as simple as a pair of eyeglasses. With the proper corrective lens, a person can drive and read. Without the glasses, they can barely walk the streets of their neighborhoods. Persons with a chronic disease are most satisfied with their health when their care is coordinated.

ACA Title III rewards coordinated health care. There is no distinction between public and private hospitals. The ACA continues financing of the teaching and safety net mission of public hospitals. The ACA decreases the size of the funding in anticipation of new funds from the expansion of Medicaid. The ACA achieves cost saving by rewarding coordinated care. Any health care business that cannot operate in the new coordinated era will not survive. Another way of thinking about coordination is through integration of sites for health care. Integration is both *horizontal* and *vertical*. *Horizontal* integration means that independent players come together to form a single organization. With this strategy, they gain an edge. Savings from the collaboration of independents can be used to invest in new technology as needed. *Vertical* integration is a fancy way of saying one-stop shopping. In an integrated environment, a person with diabetes can get laboratory tests, eye exams, and foot exams in one place. Vertical integration increases the likelihood of getting the preventive services recommended by their physician. Kaiser Permanente is an example of combined horizontal and vertical integration. They also have a niche market of service to the poor. Is the old model of a public hospital too small to operate effectively in a health care delivery market dominated by chronic disease? If safety net hospitals are to survive, what can they do to integrate? Do businesses like Ascension and Kaiser Permanente offer a vision of a delivery system that is self-sustaining *and* dedicated to public health? What are the barriers to service integration for safety net hospitals in the United States? Currently, the VHA is the only example of a public health care delivery system large enough to meet the challenges of changing disease patterns. The VHA is distributed across the United States. It achieves both patient satisfaction and cost containment by being large enough to negotiate for better prices.

Hwang and Christensen (2008) argue that the jumbled mixture of business models seen in legacy institutions prevent them from adapting. For public hospitals, what does that mean? Public hospitals are an amalgam of three basic business models. One model is a *solution shop*. A second model is a *value-adding process*. The third model is a *facilitated user network*. Solution shops are easy to understand. Public health clinics are solution shops. Think about making an appointment to see one of their doctors. You are purchasing the services of a solution shop. See the experts. Obtain their opinion. Following that advice, however, requires navigating the complex environment of health care. Part of the health disparity problem flows from inability of patients to access the solution shop. Another part of disparities flows from difficulties experienced by patients trying to follow up on the expert advice. Medical directors across these clinics are constantly working on the access problem. Attention to appointments. Control the no shows. Oversee the details that make a visit more or less efficient for the patient. All of these tasks have a place in a health care organization. These changes will not address the need for horizontal and vertical integration. The *solution shop model* does not completely explain the operation of a public health clinic. Solution shops are successful when they attract the best talent and serve clients. They function best with unlimited sums of money. Funding of public health clinics is limited in two ways. They cannot use wages and benefits as a strategy to attract the best and the brightest. They do, however, use a service-focused approach. This attracts bright people who are also dedicated to serving the poor. The limitation of client resources and the unstable nature of public financing also create barriers for public health clinics trying to adapt to the chronic disease environment.

Some public health care delivery systems use a *value-adding process business* approach to overcome the limitations of the solution shop model. Think of it as a business within a business. Any portion of health care that can be standardized is a potential value-adding process. One example of value-adding processes is the Stanford Self-Management Programs (http://patienteducation.stanford.edu/programs/). These *chronic disease self-management programs* are designed to improve the physical and emotional health of participants while reducing health care costs. The Living a Healthy Life with Chronic Conditions is one example of their workshops. It is being used by a number of public health clinics across the United States. A combination of federal (AHRQ) and state (tobacco settlement) funds financed the development of the workshops. ACA Section 3502 provides financing for primary care practices to establish a *patient-centered medical home*. The structure of a medical home is designed to deliver better care at a lower cost. The patient-centered medical home has the potential to change public health care delivery systems from complicated, expensive products into simple, affordable ones.

A third business model is a *facilitated user network*. This model harnesses the full power of collective action. Catholic Health Partners, Ascension Health, Kaiser Permanente, and the VHA are all facilitated user networks. Clients participating in these networks deposit their payments into a collective pool. The payment for care is taken from the pool. By linking outpatient and inpatient care, the cost of transition between sites is lower. Patient satisfaction with quality of care is higher. Each of these networks uses electronic health records to accomplish this linkage. They employ other strategies as well. At critical periods in their history, each network got the financing needed to expedite linkage between multiple sites of care. Catholic Health Partners and Ascension each obtained financing through its philanthropic arm. Kaiser's structure capitalizes on the healthy worker effect. Financing for growth is available from the premiums of large numbers of enrollees with few or no chronic conditions. The VHA finances its system with taxpayer dollars. Each of these networks is large enough to absorb the high costs of complex illness. Individual public hospitals are too small to support the large number of patients with chronic medical conditions. The ACA is silent on the issue of facilitated user networks of safety net hospitals. The AHRQ has been in the business of developing facilitated user networks in outpatient care since the 1980s. Funding for the development of facilitated user networks has been unstable over the 30-year period. Many of these networks are based in public health institutions like safety net hospitals, public universities, and FQHCs. Despite this challenge, primary care practice networks have grown in quality and size.

Public institutions are an enduring part of the health care delivery system in the United States. In many ways they are as resource poor as the populations they serve. Some public hospitals do not have a stable financing base. Others have reasonable public funding, but the size of the need is growing faster than their ability to expand services. Some hospitals have lost market share because local populations are aging or moving away. Many rural and critical access hospitals are faced with the challenge of serving clients who drive 100 or more miles to obtain care. The safety net hospitals discussed in this chapter serve as training sites for physicians—their salaries paid by Medicare with *graduate medical education* funds. Whether it supplements direct service or supplements the educational mission, this strategy is insufficient to meet the demands on our public health care infrastructure. In 1947, Hill Burton provided the capital investment needed to build a new public hospital system. In 1965, Medicare provided the capital investment needed to train physicians, serve elders without resources, and stabilize critical access hospitals. The ACA includes the payment incentives that private businesses need to adapt to the new chronic disease environment. Payment incentives support needed changes to become facilitated user networks. Only private businesses have the infrastructure to make the change. Where will public hospitals get the capital investment to change their historical business models? Is it time for public hospitals to engage in integration with the private delivery systems in their geographic areas? Has the U.S. business model of segregated public and private health care become unsustainable?

## BIBLIOGRAPHY

American's Hospitals and Health Systems. "American Hospital Association Groups Urge Law Makers to Continue Level Support for Disproportionate Share Hospital Programs." Letter to Senators, Representatives, and Secretary Kathleen Sebelius rejecting reductions in DSH programs, 2, 2011, http://www.aha.org/advocacy-issues/letter/2011/110301-halo-sebelius-moe.pdf.

Anderson, Jack R. "Vital Statistics of the United States, 1992 Life Tables." National Center for Health Statistics, Department of Health and Human Services, Hyattsville, 1996.

Anderson, Robert N., and Harry M. Rosenberg. "Age Standardization of Death Rates: Implementation of the Year 2000 Standard." National Vital Statistics Reports, 17, Hyattsville, 1998.

Ascension Financial Group. "Annual Report," http://www.ascensionhealth.org/annualreport/financial-info.php.

Ascension Press Team. "Ascension Health CEO Anthony R. Tersigni Named to '100 Most Influential People in Healthcare.'" Ascension Health. http://www.ascensionhealth.org/index.php?option=com_content&view=article&id=314:ascension-health-ceo-anthony-r-tersigni-named-to-100-most-influential-people-in-healthcareq&Itemid=182.

Associated Press. "Will Safety Net Hospitals Survive Health Reform?" Published electronically September 8, 2009, http://msnbc.msn.com.

Bachrach, Deborah. "Medicaid Payment Reform: What Policymakers Need to Know about Federal Law." Policy Brief, 13, Center for Health Care Strategies, Inc., 2010.

Bachrach, Deborah. "Payment Reform: Creating a Sustainable Future for Medicaid. Center for Health Care Strategies, Inc." Policy Brief, 14, Center for Health Care Strategies, Inc., 2010.

Bayne, Bijan C., Alexandra Greeley, Kate Leeson, Charles Luband, Barbara Ravage, Gina Rollins, John Galbraith Simmons, David Tilley, and Brian Vaslag. "The Safety Net: A Public Trust. Two Centuries of Care in America's Public Hospitals." Allison Hoggee, 40, National Association of Public Hospitals and Health Systems, 2006.

Becker, Alvin, and Herbert C. Schulberg. "Phasing out State Hospitals: A Psychiatric Dilemma." *New England Journal of Medicine* 294, no. 5 (1976): 255–61. http://www.ncbi.nlm.nih.gov/pubmed/811988.

Benner, Ann C. "NIH Seeks to Break New Ground in Reducing Health Disparities." Press Release Office of the Director, 2010.

Bizjournals. "Catholic Health Partners Looks to Sell Pennsylvania Group." *Business Courier*, http://www.bizjournals.com/cincinnati/print-edition/2011/08/05/catholic-health-partners-new-focus.html.

Bovbjerg, Randall R., Barbara A. Ormond, and Vicki Chen. "State Budgets under Federal Health Reform: The Extent and Causes of Variations in Estimated Impacts." Kaiser Commission on Medicaid and the Uninsured, 46, Kaiser Family Foundation, Washington, DC, 2011.

Catholic Health Partners. "Financial Report to the Community," http://www.health-partners.org.

Cline, Jane, Kevin McCarty, Roger Sevigny, Susan Voss, Kim Holland, and Sandy Praeger. "Uniform Definitions and Standard Methodologies for Medical Loss Ratios as Required by Section 2718 of the Patient Protection and Affordable Care Act of 2010 (Letter to Kathleen Siebelius, Secretary Health and Human Services)." National Association of Insurance Commissions & Center for Insurance Research and Policy, 2010.

Dawon, Milly. "Safety Net Hospital Closures Hit Poor, Uninsured Hardest." Health Services Research, Center for Advancing Health, 2011, http://www.cfah.org/hbns/archives/getDocument.cfm?documentID=22435.

Dewan, Shaila, and Kevin Sack. "A Safety-Net Hospital Falls into Financial Crisis." *New York Times,* 2008. Published electronically January 8, 2008.

Gruber, Jonathan. "Covering the Uninsured in the United States." *Journal of Economic Literature* 46, no. 3 (2008): 571–606.

Hoovers. "Company Overview: AmeriHealth Mercy Health Plan," http://www.hoovers.com/company/AmeriHealth_Mercy_Health_Plan/rtfcrti-1.html.

Hoovers. "Company Overview: Ascension Health System," http://www.hoovers.com/company/Ascension_Health/ccxyyi-1.html.

Hoovers. "Company Overview: Catholic Health Partners," http://www.hoovers.com/company/Catholic_Health_Partners/cfyrri-1.html.

Hoovers. "Company Overview: Centene Corporation," http://www.hoovers.com/company/Centene_Corporation/rfysfri-1.html.

Hoovers. "Company Overview: Kaiser Permanente," http://www.hoovers.com/company/Kaiser_Permanente/rrttcci-1.html.

Hoovers. "Company Overview: Molina Healthcare," http://www.hoovers.com/company/Molina_Healthcare_Inc/rfkrksi-1.html.

Hoyert, D. L. "Maternal Mortality and Related Concepts." Vital and Health Statistics, 20, National Center for Health Statistics, Hyattsville, 2007.

Hwang, Jason, Clayton Christensen. "Disruptive Innovation in Health Care Delivery: A Frame Work for Business Model Innovation." *Health Affairs* 27, no. 5 (2008): 1329–35.

Ritchie, James. "Catholic Health Partners CEO: Is Bigger Really Better?" *Business Courier,* 2011. Published electronically September 25, 2011. http://www.bizjournals.com/cincinnati/blog/2011/08/catholic-health-partners-ceo-is.html.

# CHAPTER 5

## Lobbyists, Advocates, and Disparity

Lobbying is about changing public policy. I would modify this idea by saying *some* lobbyists want change. Others want to preserve the existing policy. Any policy reducing inequity will alter the status quo. An altered status quo creates new winners and losers. During the health reform debate, were there advocates with specific language targeting health care inequity? The short answer is "No." During the spring of 2009, the Senate Finance Committee invited the public to submit letters airing their views of health reform policy. More than 500 written statements were submitted. The voices of individuals, advocacy groups, and professional lobbyists weighed in for a period of almost six weeks. Did any of their letters outline a strategy for ending health care inequity? Did any group use "End Health Care Inequity Now!" as a main message? No. However, an absence of specific inequity messaging does not imply lack of advocacy. As we will see, successful advocates had legislative targets. The inclusion of maternal and newborn care as an essential benefit in Title I is an example of successful advocacy. These targets are parts of a larger strategy to end health care inequity. They also had opponents.

What is a lobbyist? How do lobbyists differ from the usual citizens making their wishes known to elected officials? Legislatively, a lobbyist is defined by professionalism. The Honest Leadership and Open Government Act of 2007 (HLOGA) requires lobbyists to report to the Clerk of the U.S. House of Representatives and the secretary of the Senate on a quarterly basis. Professionals are required to list clients, fees received, and the specific issues of activity. The HLOGA also requires semiannual reporting of campaign contributions, events that honor members of Congress, or expenditures that benefit members of Congress. In addition to the HLOGA, President Obama laid out strict lobbying limits through two executive orders and three presidential directives. In these orders, the Obama administration changed what had become the usual relationship between lobbyists and some government offices. Before these orders became effective, lobbyists were hired specifically to communicate with their former colleagues. This practice was known as a revolving door. Committee staff became lobbyists for the government relations teams of private groups. In return, lobbyists were hired as staff for government agencies and committees. The revolving door preserved existing lines of communication and prevented new ones from emerging. Obama's appointees cannot seek lobbying jobs while he is president. Lobbyists can no longer give gifts to anyone in the administration. From a legislative perspective, lobbyists are now employees of the groups they represent. These groups include corporations, trade associations, labor unions, nonprofits, religious organizations, and academic institutions.

Who is a lobbyist? Like everyone else, professional lobbyists have lives outside of their profession. As individuals, they make few or no political contributions and are not politically active. An effective lobbyist is an advocate who knows the clients' interests and the legislative process. They educate legislators about the impact of an action on the clients' interests. Academics who study lobbying say that an education, per se, does not change the behavior of a legislator. The legislator must also share the interest with the client. For the lobbyist to be successful, there are shared interests that include politics as well as policy. The effective lobbyist sells a specific legislative approach. For example, a group wants to decrease the number of persons enrolled in Medicaid. The reasons behind the opposition are irrelevant. They are out to achieve measurable declines in the number served. There are multiple strategies for lobbyists hired by the group. A lobbyist could develop a list of upcoming bills and promote a voting pattern to achieve the designed outcome. The lobbyist could draft a modification of a bill under review—again designed to achieve the desired effect. The lobbyist could develop new legislative text. It could be shopped around to obtain cosponsors. A thorough knowledge of legislative language, as well as politics and protocol, enhances the value of a lobbyist.

Were any lobbyist's requests relevant to the problem of health care inequity? Maybe, if inequity advocacy is defined as enlightened self-interest. Outside of the Washington, District of Columbia, political sphere, the image of a lobbyist looks a lot like Santa in a Brooks Brothers suit. He moves from office to office dropping off bags of money in exchange for good behavior. In this instance, the desirable behavior consists of votes for legislation leading to enhancing the profit for Santa's workshop. No matter the details, the ultimate goal is the production of legislation that increases the workshop's profitability. Meanwhile, innocents sleep and wait for the new day of improved health care. A lobbyist will work for health care inequity if it is in the client's interest to do so. Does the public have a problem with the existence of lobbyists? A Pew Center public opinion poll on January 26, 2010, showed that there is little interest in reducing the influence of lobbyists. Only 36 percent of respondents view reducing their influence in Washington as a top priority. Another 34 percent view reducing influence as important but not a priority. Most Americans view lobbyists and the process of lobbying as a means to a self-serving end, not a common good. It is not clear whether the public distinguishes between lobbying and advocacy.

What about advocates? Advocacy is the face of grassroots citizens in action. Citizens work for causes that carry the force of justice. Each year citizen groups organize visits to Congressional offices. For example, the Alzheimer's Association sponsors an all-day workshop in Washington, DC to train everyday citizens to speak with their elected officials. Spouses, children, and grandchildren living with Alzheimer's disease patients spread out across Capitol Hill. Moving from office to office, they deposit informational material. This material describes desired legislative behavior. In the interest of full disclosure, I should tell you that I have volunteered as an unpaid advocate on minority issues and older adults for the Alzheimer's Association since 1995. Sometimes we advocate for a specific vote on a single piece of legislation. In 2010, advocates celebrated the passage of Public Law 111-375. The National Alzheimer's Project Act of 2011 establishes a federal-level coordination of programs targeting Alzheimer's disease. Other times, we provide information about the widespread nature of Alzheimer's disease. A similar process is employed by advocacy groups as diverse as the American Heart Association, the National Association of Community Health Centers, and the American College of Nurse-Midwives. As practiced, advocacy is viewed as an honorable process for collective action. Advocates are not lobbyists. Or are they? Are lobbyists the mischievous cousin of advocates? Is the mischief defined by policies or tactics used to promote legislation? Both work to influence legislative processes. During the ACA debate, advocates and lobbyists played a significant role in the final content of ACA. Advocates wanted increased access to health care for their group or disease. Lobbyists wanted expanded access as well or to prevent their current share from being cut. The primary difference was that lobbyists' were paid for their time and talents. Advocates viewed their cause through a personal lens.

The letters to congressional committees from advocates and lobbyists are publically available through Freedom of Information Act requests. Many letters are also available on the advocate's website. Letter writing is an inexpensive way to communicate with legislators. The Senate Finance Committee, for example, received thousands of letters and e-mails during the health care reform debate. If there is a common message in these letters, it is "Health reform: what's in it for me?" With the possible exception of the Children's Defense Fund, the messages are not specific to the issue of inequity. The following list shows a group and a one sentence summary of their message. Both the italics and language belongs to me:

Alzheimer's Association: *"Our vision is a world without Alzheimer's disease."*

American Heart Association: *"Health reform: if it isn't affordable, it isn't fixed."*

American Medical Association: "This is certainly not the bill we would have written, but we cannot let the perfect be the enemy of the good."

National Association of Community Health Centers: *"Health center advocacy is the key to our future!"*

Children's Defense Fund: *"Get health coverage for all children."*

What about minority-focused civil rights groups such as the National Association for the Advancement of Colored People (NAACP) and the National Council of La Raza? The National Council of La Raza's message was *"health care reform, health care for all."* In a postcard campaign targeting Latinos throughout the United States, the National Council of La Raza was able to deliver this message to the Congress requesting health care reform legislation consisting of quality, affordable health care for all. The campaign consisted of a postcard sent to the elected official that read:

I need quality health care for my family and community.

*Necesito buen cuidado di salud para mi familia y mi comunidad.*

The National Association for the Advancement of Colored People has a concept of health care inequity that is explicitly stated in element three shown later. This is not the kind of messaging that moves people to march. It is complex. Inequity is sandwiched between insurance issues like coverage, benefits, and choice. Still, it is there. The following is a sampling of the message from the National Association for the Advancement of Colored People (NAACP) website:

> The NAACP is committed to eliminating the racial and ethnic disparities in our health care system that plague people of color in the United States . . . the NAACP is working hard to ensure that the final product has the following four elements: (1) *full health care coverage that is affordable* to every individual, family, and business which also provides coverage for pre-existing conditions; (2) *standard, comprehensive health care benefits* that meet everyone's needs from preventive to chronic care; (3) *equity in health care access*, treatment, research, and resources to all Americans, including communities of color, and stronger, more comprehensive health services in low income communities; and (4) the *choice* of a private (allowing recipients to stay with their existing health care coverage if they choose) or public health care plan, which includes a new public health care plan (the "public option").

Health care advocacy is not new. History shows that skilled advocacy is effective when paired with a goal perceived as being righteous. History also shows the composition, timing, and strategies for advocacy are different when the interests of America's minorities are involved. The personal wealth and influence of the voices involved drives the success of advocacy in general. However, advocates for minority-related issues have the extra requirement to justify their advocacy. Is a particular disease really a problem for the minority group? In addition to advocacy for the disease, activists with an interest in a specific group also had to lobby for the collection of public health data. These groups have made the case that insufficient data is a form of health care inequity. Consider the problem of cancer deaths among Asians in the United States. As a group, Asians have the highest life expectancy of any racial or ethnic group in the United States. At every age, their risk of dying is significantly lower than other groups—whites included. However, cancer is the leading cause of death for middle-aged and older Asians. From the national perspective, cancer is not a public health problem for Asians. From the perspective of Japanese Americans, cancer deaths are a big problem. The Centers for Disease Control and Prevention began to collect statistics on race and ethnicity starting in the 1980s. Before then, the data needed to see the suffering of Asians with cancer was not available. The larger community of public health workers and advocates are beginning to understand the nuances of disease and geography. *Scientific advocacy*, that is, the use of public health data to justify a request, is a relatively new tactic. Some advocates could tell a compelling story about a single individual and be heard. The powers of stories told by minority advocates were discounted. Racial stereotypes created barriers in the minds of legislators. Advocacy for cancer in the United States has historical roots. Its history shows the different requirements for activism on behalf of an ethnic group.

The American Cancer Society combines skilled advocacy and a righteous goal. The American Cancer Society emphasizes its community basis. It harnesses the free labor of volunteers who have direct experience with cancer. The American Cancer Society is dedicated to *eliminating* cancer and the suffering it causes. The American Cancer Society is a not-for-profit organization. Its roots can be traced back to 1912 with a story about Mary Lasker's maid. Mrs. Lasker's story was simple. Her maid died because there was no cancer treatment available. The advocacy of Mrs. Lasker and others led Congress to pass the National Cancer Act of 1937. Once signed by President Roosevelt, it established the National Cancer Institute. Congress started the National Cancer Institute with an appropriation of 700,000 dollars each fiscal year to support cancer research. This appropriation was dwarfed by the fund-raising efforts of ACS volunteers. The first American Cancer Society fund-raising campaign in 1945 earned more than four million dollars. Twenty-five percent was set aside for research. Since the federal government was spending only a total of 750,000 dollars for cancer research during the same year, the amount raised by the American Cancer Society was significant. The donations obtained by American Cancer Society are many times that today. The *Relay for Life* program raised 60 million dollars in 2010. The American Cancer Society has also played a role guiding the overall direction of cancer science through its director of research. In 2007, the American Cancer Society allocated 17 percent of its donations to research (2008 Internal Revenue Service Form 990). The American Cancer Society makes this report available online. Fifty-eight percent of donations were allocated to patient support, treatment, and detection. A persistent focus by advocates has created stability for the support of cancer research and the care of cancer patients. While advocacy draws attention to a disease, it risks diversion of resources from the larger issue of health care for illness. With every action, there are consequences. Do advocates create inequity with their single focus? Is inequity an unsuspected product of single-issue advocacy?

The strategies used by advocates to move politicians are not well documented. For example, the war on cancer was inadvertently launched in 1969 when President Richard M. Nixon tried to reduce the budget of the National Cancer Institute. We do not know the details surrounding his conversion from budget reductionist to funder-in-chief. By 1971, Nixon declared war on cancer during his January State of the Union address:

> I will also ask for an appropriation of an extra One hundred million dollars to launch an intensive campaign to find a cure for cancer, and I will ask later for whatever additional funds can effectively be used. The time has come in America when the same kind of concentrated effort that split the atom and took man to the moon should be turned toward conquering this dread disease. Let us make a total national commitment to achieve this goal.

On December 23, 1971, President Nixon signed the National Cancer Act of 1971 (Public Law 92-218). For U.S. minority groups, this act started a National Cancer Program. The act improved the cancer data of the state and health care agencies. Before the existence of these data, some researchers argued that minorities did not experience cancer to the same extent as whites. With the National Cancer Act, the era of data-based scientific advocacy had begun. Like the 1937 law, the National Cancer Act of 1971 was singularly focused on cancer.

The ACA contains sections requiring hospitals to collect data on patient characteristics such as race, ethnicity, primary language, and disability. A common thread throughout health care delivery advocacy in the United States is the need for data—particularly for minority groups. U.S. policies mandating the collection of health statistics data have their own evolving history. This history begins in the 1930s. The availability of treatments for infectious diseases after World War II created a demand for health statistics data. The development and diffusion of a national system for the collection of mortality data gave rise to our current vital statistics of the U.S. accounting system. With these data, public health officials can monitor the changing causes of death, providing snapshots of regional variation. Without a vital statistics system, the nation would not be able to identify disease outbreaks. We take this system for granted. It did not become functional in all states until 1950. Without data, the public health sector could not see the cancer illness and deaths. Once the vital statistics system was established, there were still structural barriers to documenting health care inequity. Categories for racial and ethnic groups were absent. In national surveys as late as the 1970s, participants were labeled as white and nonwhite. African Americans, Mexican Americans, and Asian Americans lived in the United States during the 1950s. The vital statistics system, however, did not see them. The Indian Health Service was fully operational during the development of the vital statistics system. However, data from the Indian Health Service was not incorporated into the system. The Centers for Disease Control and Prevention (CDC) routinely monitor vital statistics for census-defined categories of racial and ethnic groups. The barrier between the Indian Health Service and the vital statistics system persists to this day. It is still impossible to see the health care quality, disease burden, and mortality experience of Indian Health Service users *within the context* of the larger U.S. health care delivery system.

Throughout U.S. history, there has been advocacy to eliminate segregation in the health care delivery system. Although President Franklin Roosevelt was viewed fondly by blacks during the Great Depression, New Deal health care policies did nothing to alter the strict segregation of U.S. hospitals. While Social Security was enacted to provide pension and disability benefits, it excluded domestic servants. These workers were primarily females from minority and immigrant groups—two groups experiencing care inequity. The combined impact of Hill Burton (1947) and Medicare (1965) created financial incentives to eliminate segregation in hospitals. The development of financial incentives through payment policies is a strategy that advocates have employed repeatedly to open health care access.

Effective advocacy for the cancer care of African Americans was initiated with the resources available through the National Cancer Act of 1971. This is almost 30 years after Mrs. Lasker's advocacy for the National Cancer Institute. A group of professors from Howard University's College of Medicine led a national coalition to use the new vital statistics data to illustrate excess cancer mortality and its link with poverty. Before their analyses, the scientific literature of the day argued that cancer was not a problem for blacks. The public health community argued that cancer was not an issue because it did not appear in their data. The advocates countered with the argument that if it is not measured, how can you know? In 1978, the American Cancer Society elected its first African American president, LaSalle Leffall, a leader of the Howard group. Another member, Harold Freeman, became American Cancer Society president in 1998. Unlike the 1912 American Cancer Society founders, neither man had great family wealth. Both relied on *scientific advocacy*. This form of advocacy uses vital statistics data to show disease patterns. They built a coalition of African Americans including physicians, researchers, and public health officials. In scientific conferences, meetings, and research journals they spoke truth to power. Power included governmental agencies, professional medical groups, and health care industry leaders. Unfortunately, we do not have a detailed record of their advocacy process. Their work led to legislation creating the Office of Minority Health and Health Disparities within the Centers for Disease Control (Public Law 103–43). This act also expanded breast cancer control efforts and mandated inclusion of women and minorities in National Institutes of Health–funded research. Their advocacy also led to increased access to training of minority scientists. Opening the National Cancer Institute forced an initiative across multiple National Institutes of Health units to train minority researchers. Minority cancer advocacy of the 1970s is an example of single issue advocacy opening multiple barriers. The impact of science-based advocacy by minority professionals on the direction of all medical research funding continues. Enhanced research funding created financial incentives for university-based researchers to actively recruit African Americans, Hispanics, and Asians into clinical studies. The Minority Health and Health Disparities Research and Education Act of 2000 (Public Law 106–525) established a National Center on Minority Health and Health Disparities. With the passage of the ACA, this center became a fully fledged NIH National Institute on Minority Health and Health Disparities (Section 10334).

Racial and ethnic groups were not the only group systematically excluded from medical research. Older adults were systematically excluded from all clinical trials—not just cancer treatment trials. Prior to 2000, only 25 percent of patients enrolled in clinical trials were aged 65 and older. Clinical trials are the vetting process for all treatments used in the United States. Vital statistics data shows that 63 percent of all patients with cancer are older adults. Systematic exclusion of older adults created physicians blind to the true risks and benefits of the medications used for routine cancer treatment. This disparity was overcome with advocacy by the American Cancer Society. The American Cancer Society and the Southwest Oncology Group launched a campaign to change the Medicare payment policies that created barriers to participation in clinical trials. The primary policy change involved payment for routine care costs associated with the trial. Before 2000, trial participants paid a portion of costs associated with the trials *out of their own pockets*. The reader should understand that participation in clinical trials is a strategy that many patients use to gain access to the latest cancer treatments. It is a tactic used to prolong life during late-stage disease. The requirement to pay medical costs created access barriers for low-income older adults. Advocates helped President Bill Clinton and Congress understand this economic barrier to advanced cancer care. On June 7, 2000, President Clinton issued an executive memorandum directing the Secretary of the Health and Human Services to "explicitly authorize [Medicare] payment for routine patient care costs . . . and costs due to medical complications associated with participation in clinical trials." The Centers for Medicare and Medicaid Services responded to the executive order with the clinical trial policy national coverage determination (NCD) issued on September 19, 2000. This policy increased the participation of all Medicare beneficiaries in cancer clinical trials. Treatments are now evaluated for their safety and effectiveness specifically with older adults. The strategy by advocates to influence payment policy has increased the safety of treatments for older adults. Advocates for children engaged in a similar process. Children are less likely to enroll in a clinical trial for many reasons. The ability of their parents to pay for trial-related health care costs is one of them. The net result of this economic barrier is that medicines given to children are not completely evaluated for their safety and effectiveness. The Pediatric Exclusivity Provision of the Food and Drug Administration's (FDA) Modernization Act of 1997 became law under the Best Pharmaceuticals for Children Act (BPCA) in 2002. The BPCA gives drug manufacturers a voluntary incentive of an additional six months of marketing exclusivity and the ability to sell their drug without competition from generic drugs. This exclusivity is the reward for conducting studies of drugs that FDA determines may be useful to children. The Pediatric Rule was passed as the Pediatric Research Equity Act (PREA) in 2003. PREA authorizes FDA to require manufacturers of new drug and biologic products to conduct pediatric studies in certain circumstances. Together, these two acts have encouraged the development of important new information for drugs used to treat children. In the United States, linking financial incentives with policies that promote inclusion is an advocacy strategy to lower barriers in the health care delivery system for minorities, elders, and children.

Infant and maternal mortality in the United States is a public health issue. The likelihood that a woman or infant will die during the birthing process is higher than one would expect. This excess risk is true for all women from all racial and ethnic groups living in the United States. The rates are still higher for African American and Native American women. There is a large collection of reports linking delayed maternity care with this unacceptable outcome. During the development of the ACA, advocates worked to promote policies to facilitate access during the earliest stages of pregnancy. The advocacy surrounding maternity care illustrates the full range of opinions, tactics, and messaging during the development of the ACA. For women in all racial and ethnic groups, access to maternity care is a health care inequity issue. The problem and its resolution cannot be explained in the 15-second sound bites favored by media. Policy to improve access for pregnant women is complex. To improve access, structural changes to both public and private insurance plans were needed. Advocates had to be smart about each corner of the health insurance market. Why? First, there is a rigid separation within U.S. health insurance markets. In the United States, almost 70 percent of women of reproductive age are covered by employer-sponsored health insurance plans. Some women are covered by a comprehensive plan. Others have a job, but their employer's plan places limits on maternity care. Still others have a job but no employer-sponsored insurance. These are the health care inequities faced by women in the workplace. Some advocates focused on correcting the inequities created by employer-sponsored plans. The ACA Title I Essential Benefit Provision is an outgrowth of this advocacy.

For unemployed women or those living in low-income families, there is Medicaid, the public insurance plan. Medicaid pays for at least 4 in 10 births in the United States. During 2008, the percentage of births covered by Medicaid ranged from a low of 23 percent in New Hampshire to a high of 63 percent in Louisiana. In many states, eligibility for Medicaid is defined by an income ceiling. At this point, it may occur to you to ask: "How can a person have a job and not have health insurance to cover maternity care?" Medicaid is just one silo in the hypersegmented health insurance markets. Prior to enactment of the ACA, there was no federal requirement to cover maternity care. Individual, small, and employer-sponsored markets did not uniformly offer any maternity care. When it was offered, the details of benefits were wide ranging. Some advocates focused on the inequities created by state-to-state variation in Medicaid eligibility. Their handiwork can be seen in Title II policies.

Maternity care policy advocates did not have a single goal. There was a barrage of confusing policies aimed at legislators. All advocates promised cost savings. Each policy was linked to a financial incentive. Each policy was linked to a single insurance market, sometimes public, sometimes private. This helped to simplify messaging during debates. Increasing access was a common thread in most messages. However, others opposed any change. Enhancing Medicaid was the most common policy among advocates. Opponents wanted to limit the access of immigrants to Medicaid. There were advocates for private insurance market issues. Making maternity care an *essential benefit* for all plans was a popular approach. Opponents objected to insurance premiums that included costs for care that they did not need. For each side, there were no explicit references to health care inequity.

There is a long history of advocacy for pregnant women in the workplace. Its history is as complex as the one surrounding cancer, health data, and clinical trials. There have been two major pieces of legislation in the past 40 years designed to stabilize civil rights for pregnant women in the workplace. A prime goal of each was preserving the jobs of pregnant women. Prior to these laws, employers commonly fired pregnant women. In 1978, the Congress amended Title VII of the Civil Rights Act with the Pregnancy Discrimination Act. It made discrimination on the basis of pregnancy, childbirth, or related medical conditions unlawful, declaring it a form of sex discrimination. This law covers only employers with 15 or more employees. It required equal coverage of illnesses for pregnant and nonpregnant employees. It did not require employer-sponsored health insurance plans to provide maternity care as an insurance benefit. Employers supplied maternity benefits as a perk for their married, male workers to support their families. In the 1960s and 1970s, women were just beginning to enter the workforce in large numbers. By the 1990s, employer-sponsored plans began to limit pregnancy coverage as a strategy to control health care costs. Consider the following story:

> A few weeks after my first prenatal exam, I got a letter from my health insurance company. It informed me that my pregnancy would not be covered because I wasn't insured at the time of conception. The fact that I did not know that I was pregnant at the time of my conception was irrelevant. I had a complicated pregnancy with preeclampsia, which raised my blood pressure and caused my kidneys to function poorly. Because I required a month of hospitalization and numerous tests, the costs were exorbitant. But I was fortunate. My baby was healthy and my previous insurance company paid the initial bills through the waiting period. . . . What about all the women who are not as lucky as I am?

Enacted in 1996, the Health Insurance Portability and Accountability Act prevented group plans from considering pregnancy a preexisting condition. It ended the practice of excluding coverage for prenatal care. Before

Health Insurance Portability and Accountability Act, insurance plans could refuse to pay for prenatal care and only pay for the expenses associated with birth. Separating prenatal care from actual birth care is strictly a business model and not a medical one. Again, Health Insurance Portability and Accountability Act rules applied to only group plans with maternity coverage. Health Insurance Portability and Accountability Act did not require employer-sponsored health insurance plans to provide maternity care as an insurance benefit. Until the ACA health insurance policy standards become law in 2014, employed women will not be protected from this experience.

Maternity care caused a variety of groups to emerge. Some advocates based their policy on moral grounds. Others use scientific advocacy and public health statistics. Opponents raised concerns about cost of care. There were nasty debates about the use of these services by illegal immigrants. Readers who are interested in specific maternity care policies are encouraged to refer Public Law 111-148:

Section 1302: Essential health benefits requirement.

Section 2202: Hospitals to make presumptive eligibility determination for Medicaid.

Section 2301: Coverage for free-standing birth center services.

Section 2801: Medicaid and CHIP Payment and Access Commission assessment of policies affecting all Medicaid beneficiaries.

Section 2951: Maternal, infant, and early childhood home visiting programs.

Section 4302: Understanding health disparities—data collection and analysis. These data will have a specific application to measuring changes in maternal and infant deaths.

To fully link tactics and advocacy, let us examine two groups: The March of Dimes (TMD) and their opponents in the Republican Party—Senator Jon Kyl (R-Arizona), Tom Coburn (R-Oklahoma), and James Walsh, a blogger for *NewsMax*. TMD is one of the most successful and well-known nonprofit foundations in the United States. The mission of TMD is to improve the health of babies by preventing birth defects and infant mortality. It was founded in 1938 to fight polio. After polio was controlled by the invention of a vaccine, TMD turned its efforts to eradicating birth defects. To date, TMD has raised more than almost two billion dollars to fund research and programs to prevent premature birth. The foundation funds research, giving grants to hundreds of scientists annually at a cost of more than 20 million dollars. It organizes fund-raising events to promote awareness and bring in cash for its programs. It helps run community services and educational projects. TMD is responsible for backing major scientific breakthroughs in genetics and prenatal health. The organization has been highly effective in advocating for women's and children's health. A legislative success in the 1980s was the elimination of the drive by maternity stay. This legislation guaranteed women a minimum hospital stay of 48 hours after giving birth to a baby. TMD has been cited as an example of bureaucracy because it did not disband after it achieved its mission of eliminating polio in the 1950s. The organization's new mission, "to improve the health of babies by preventing birth defects, premature birth, and infant mortality," may justify its existence indefinitely.

In their advocacy letter to the Senate Finance Committee, TMD describes the maternity care barriers created by employer-sponsored insurance plans. Almost 200 million persons in the United States obtain their health insurance through employer-sponsored plans. This covers almost 70 percent of women in their reproductive years. TMD describes the barrier to maternity care created by private insurance plans:

> The March of Dimes supports the proposal to prohibit the exclusion of coverage for pre-existing health conditions for all insurance plans in the non-group, micro group and small group markets, and in the health insurance exchange. Given that one in five women of child-bearing age [or] twelve million is uninsured (according to United States Census Bureau data) and that fifty percent of pregnancies are unplanned, the current practice of treating pregnancy as a pre-existing condition has made it impossible for many pregnant women to obtain affordable health coverage for maternity care. Removing this barrier to coverage is an important component of health reform.

TMD supports the proposal to require all health insurance plans in the nongroup, micro group, and small group markets, and in the health insurance exchange to cover maternity and newborn care. A 2006 Georgetown University study commissioned by TMD found that 19 states had adopted laws to require coverage of maternity care. In states without such requirements, maternity coverage was typically not available in the individual and small group markets. A federal standard to ensure that maternity coverage is available to all women, regardless of where they live, is essential as part of health reform. ACA Title I, Section 1302 makes maternity care a standard benefit.

A universal health insurance benefit to cover maternity care would seem like mom and apple pie. Who would be opposed to this policy? There were opponents. Consider the following exchange between Senator Jon Kyl (R-Arizona) and Senator Debbie Stabenow (D-Michigan). Just before the Senate Finance Committee wrapped up for the long weekend, members debated one of Kyl's amendments in striking language that defined employer benefits. Senator Debbie Stabenow (D-Michigan) argues that insurers must cover basic maternity care:

> "I don't need maternity care," Kyl said. "So requiring that on my insurance policy is something that I don't need and will make the policy more expensive."
>
> Stabenow interrupted: "I think your mom probably did."

The silence in the hearing room was broken with snickers and chuckles. The amendment was defeated by a margin of 9 to 14 and the meeting was adjourned. In addition to Jon Kyl, most Republican members of the Senate Finance Committee voted against including maternity care as a basic benefit.

Advocacy activity during the ACA was focused on a policy called *presumptive eligibility* (PE). The final version of ACA Title II, Section 2202 allows hospitals to make PE determination for Medicaid. What is PE? In their letter to the Senate Finance Committee, TMD advocates strongly for this policy:

> The March of Dimes also recommends that states be required to implement presumptive eligibility for all pregnant women and children in Medicaid and CHIP. . . . Experience has demonstrated that presumptive eligibility increases the proportion of pregnant women on Medicaid who receive early prenatal care.

Why does an organization like TMD need to advocate for this seemingly obscure policy? Oklahoma Medicaid illustrates PE in action. Oklahoma Medicaid uses PE to provide care for pregnant women before a formal determination of eligibility. A nurse or physician can assume for one or two visits that the woman is eligible. PE encourages pregnant women to seek prenatal care early in their pregnancy rather than waiting several weeks for administrative clearance. PE also ensures payment to qualified providers for the prenatal care. Eligibility determination often takes several months. PE provides support during the review process. As long as the provider has evidence that the net family income of the pregnant woman does not exceed 185 percent of the FPL, the provider can treat under PE and get paid for the service.

Embedded within the opposition to PE is a concern about immigrant access to health care. Senator Tom Coburn (R-Oklahoma), an obstetrician, opposed the policy of PE:

> "Presumptive eligibility" is the idea that anyone who shows up at a hospital or doctor's office is presumed to be eligible for Medicaid. These provisions are not only budget-busters, but both are loopholes designed for defrauding the system that could allow illegal aliens or anyone else to get health care paid for by taxpayers, whether or not they are truly eligible and in need.

James Walsh, a blogger for *NewsMax,* presented the common form of the advocacy against PE:

> What provisions will the awaited "health insurance reform" bill have for legal and illegal aliens? The final bill may declare no free health care for aliens, legal or illegal, just as Section 246 of the Pelosi-Waxman bill does. Like the Pelosi-Waxman bill, however, the final bill probably will have sections that prohibit discrimination, that leave determination of eligibility to Obama bureaucrats, and that include *presumptive eligibility.* If contested, litigators for presumptive eligibility will cite the Equal Protection Clause of the United States Constitution to assure access to Obama care for legal and illegal aliens.

PE has the ability to lower barriers to care. A lower barrier to maternity care has a clear link to infant mortality. TMD, however, does not present a message combining these two ideas. Instead, TMD has messages directly advocating a need for better data to measure racial disparities:

> Significant racial disparities exist among maternal . . . outcomes. Women of color and their children face great challenges in obtaining needed health care as well as devastating health effects that can result from lack of access to care. In 2007, thirty seven percent of Hispanic women of child bearing age and twenty four percent of non-Hispanic black women of child bearing age were uninsured

according to figures prepared by the United States Census Bureau. The national average is nearly twenty percent. As noted above and documented by the Institute of Medicine of the National Academies, uninsured pregnant women have a difficult time accessing maternity care. Approximately twenty five percent of black and Hispanic pregnant women did not get prenatal care in the first three months of pregnancy. The national average is sixteen percent without care in the first three months.

TMD also recognized the needs of legal immigrants. Current law required this group to wait for five years before becoming eligible for Medicaid-supported health care. TMD is an advocate that clearly voices a health equity agenda. It just does not explicitly state it. This has direct consequences for pregnant women and children:

> The March of Dimes supports improving the collection of health disparities data for the Medicaid and CHIP populations. In addition, the March of Dimes strongly supports eliminating the five year waiting period for non-pregnant adult legal immigrants. This policy will help expand access to coverage for women of child bearing age.

To sort through the noise surrounding health care reform, let us return to the original question: Did TMD use *ending health care inequity* as a main message? No. Did TMD promote three useful policies? Perhaps it did. The link between inequity, *presumptive eligibility,* and *essential benefit* is obvious only to policy wonks. If you know Medicaid, you know the use of PE. If you understand private insurance markets, you know the impact of maternity exclusion clauses. TMD also advocated for improved data. Section 4302 is clearly linked to the request for improved health disparity data in Medicaid and CHIP populations. If you know about the five-year waiting period for Medicaid, you understand barriers to care confronting legal immigrants to the United States. In the final analysis, TMD *did* advocate for policies with direct impact on health care inequity. TMD does not use the language of civil rights. It uses the language of insurance reform.

## SUMMARY

There is no straight path through policy when your goal is elimination of health care inequity. Activists for specific policies usually do not think through the downstream consequences. Most are volunteers. These volunteers have a personal experience with the problem at hand. Some have experienced difficulty obtaining care while pregnant. Some have experience with fighting insurance companies for benefits. Others have witnessed the death of a loved one. In the current climate, the energy of volunteers is being harnessed by formal organizations that are dedicated to one problem. Alzheimer's disease, cancer, maternal and child issues are just a few of the causes that move individuals to action. The formal organizations measure their impact by various means. Does the organization have a large number of volunteers? Are the volunteers active, that is, are there a number of fund-raising events? How much money is donated during the event? Can we move legislators to act on the behalf of our cause? How many patients are supported with the resources generated by the volunteers? These are all good endpoints. There are no formal organizations with a singular focus on health care inequities.

Health care inequities are a manifestation of the larger issue of civil rights. There are a number of civil rights–focused organizations. Without a formal organization, there are no groups with a core mission of ending health disparities. Without a formal organization, there are no volunteers, no solicitation of funding, and no targeted legislative advocacy. In our system, it also means that there is no coherent policy analysis. There are think tanks like the Center for American Progress, Center for Health System Change, Kaiser Family Foundation, Robert Wood Johnson Foundation, the Commonwealth Fund, and the Urban Institute. Health disparities are a sidebar to their larger agenda to promote social progress. The federal government has created an institutional home to work on the problem of minority health through the creation of the National Institute on Minority Health and Health Disparities (NIMHD). The ACA contained legislative language to give NIMHD a defined role in the National Institute of Health's agenda against disparities. This new structure is a welcome advance. It will certainly integrate health disparities into the research enterprise. Its director, Dr. John Ruffin, will act as the primary federal official with responsibility for coordinating this research activity. He represents the next generation of scientific advocacy. He has a platform to influence the direction of health disparity research. This function is similar to one performed by the scientific director of the ACS or the Alzheimer's Association. Unlike the advocacy groups, NIMHD is a governmental agency. It cannot send legions of volunteers to walk the halls of Congress or individual state houses influencing legislative action. The Joint Center for Political and Economic Studies is an advocacy group that played a central role in the health disparity debate. As articulated by Ralph Everett, president and CEO, their central mission is "building relationships across racial and ethnic lines in order to strengthen the nation's pluralistic society . . ." There is a unit dedicated to Health Policy within the Joint Center. It is led by Brian Smedley. Like the parent organization, the Health Policy Institute of the Joint Center is a solutions shop. It has been very effective in bringing together community leaders across the country. Their efforts are focused on the connection between one's neighborhood and health equity. This strategy, like NIMHD, represents the next generation of scientific advocacy. Is there evidence of grassroots advocacy on the problem of health disparity?

Ultimately, grassroots advocates are required to shape the local changes leading to equitable health care. During the debate surrounding health care reform, advocacy was largely focused on insurance, health care delivery systems, and payment reforms. How can advocates connect these three policy processes to health disparities? The answer to this question links grassroots advocacy to ACA policy. Equity and parity are sensed at the local level. It is a day-to-day encounter with the local institutions. Did you get what you came for? Does it feel right? Since all health care is local, the resolution of the barriers that create health care inequity will occur at the local level. Are there tools in the ACA that can be used by local advocates? After all, federal policy operates at the 50,000-foot level where individuals are lumped into categories. Individuals become members of an employer-sponsored plan. Individuals are described as beneficiaries in a public health insurance plan. The hospitals, physician offices, and other sites of care are lumped into a single category called health care delivery systems. At the federal level, each individual, employer, and health care delivery system is the same. The 50,000-foot federal view creates a frame of reference for national discussion. Threads that are common to all areas are clearly seen. Without this perspective, the needed quality improvement processes legislated in Title III would never have been crafted. National quality improvement strategies could not be coordinated.

Grassroots activists can play a role in local cost containment efforts. When local groups participate in the quality improvement process, the cost control efforts are less harsh. Grassroots activism gives local officials alternatives to making straight percentage cuts in programs. *Money Follows the Person* is a demonstration program initially authorized in Section 6071 of the Deficit Reduction Act of 2005. It was designed to help states with the portion of their Medicaid budgets spent on long-term care. Each state is facing the problem of cutting Medicaid funds. The Money Follows the Person demonstration gives each state the opportunity to craft a local strategy to guide the Medicaid cutbacks. This approach humanizes cost control measures by honoring the fundamental desire of disabled persons to stay in their communities. Institutional care is more expensive and less satisfactory than services brought into the home. Each jurisdiction will need local participation as the process for delivering these services is developed. In some areas of the United States, advocates for affordable housing are coming together with advocates for the disabled to develop locally sustainable solutions. This is how advocacy for the health equity provisions of ACA moves out of the 50,000-foot level. In every instance, putting ACA policy into practice happens between the 5-foot to 5,000-foot level. There are local supporters and opponents for the ACA. Their reasons for support or opposition can be completely different from those expressed in the national debate. Local politics add another layer. Without organized grassroots groups dedicated to the problem of health equity, there is no local advocacy. The ACA provided tools for local advocacy. To use these tools, advocates will need to educate themselves. The Joint Center for Political and Economic Studies is a national organization that has already begun the process of educating local advocates with their Place and Health Equity program. More programs like this one are needed.

## BIBLIOGRAPHY

American Hospital Association. "Comments to the Senate Finance Committee on Expanding Health Care Coverage: Proposals to Provide Affordable Coverage to All Americans," May 21, 2009.

Avitzur, Orly. "When Health Insurance Won't Cover Your Pregnancy." *Consumer Reports Health*, 2008, http://news.consumerreports.org/health/2008/08/when-health-ins.html.

Baumgartner, Frank R., Jeffrey M. Berry, Marie Hojnacki, David C. Kimball, and Beth L. Leech. *Lobbying and Policy Change: Who Wins, Who Loses, and Why*. Chicago: University of Chicago Press, 2009.

Byrd, W. Michael, and Linda A. Clayton. *An American Health Dilemma: Race, Medicine, and Health Care in the United States 1900-2000*. New York: Routledge, 2002.

Claxton, Gary, Biance DiJulio, Benjamin Finder, Janet Lundy, Megan McHugh, Awo Osei-Anto, Heidi Whitmore, Jeremy Pickreign, and Jon Gabel. "Employer Health Benefits: 2009 Summary of Findings." Kaiser Family Foundation, Health Research & Education Trust, National Opinion Research Center, 2009.

Congressional Research Office. "The Health Insurance Portability and Accountability Act (HIPAA) of 1996: Overview and Guidance on Frequently Asked Questions."

Cossman, J. S., W. L. James, A. G. Cosby, and R. E. Cossman. "Underlying Causes of the Emerging Nonmetropolitan Mortality Penalty." *American Journal of Public Health* 100, no. 8 (2010): 1417–19.

Dominitz, Jason A., Charles Maynard, Kevin G. Billingsley, and Edward J. Boyko. "Race, Treatment, and Survival of Veterans with Cancer of the Distal Esophagus and Gastric Cardia." *Medical Care* 40, no. 1, Supplement: Racial-disparities research in Veterans Healthcare Administration (2002): I14–I26.

Eggen, Dan, and R. Jeffrey Smith. "Lobbying Rules Surpass Those of Previous Presidents, Experts Say." *Washington Post,* 2009. Published electronically January 22, 2009. http://www.washingtonpost.com/wp-dyn/content/article/2009/01/21/AR2009012103472.html.

Epstein, Ronald M., Brian S. Alper, and Timothy E. Quill. "Communicating Evidence for Participatory Decision Making." *Journal of the American Medical Association* 291, no. 19 (2004): 2359–66.

Faquet, Guy B. *The War on Cancer: An Anatomy of Failure, a Blueprint for the Future.* New York: Springer, 2005.

Gannon, Frank. "5.11.71: RN Urges Congressional Passage of National Cancer Act." The Richard Nixon Foundation, http://blog.nixonfoundation.org/2011/05/5-11-71-rn-urges-congressional-passage-of-his-proposed-legislation-to-establish-a-national-cancer-program/.

Ghazal, Maria. "Rin 0938-Aq17 Comments Re: Proposed Rule for Medicare Program; Availability of Medicare Data for Performance Measurement (June 8, 2011)." 5: *Business Roundtable,* 2011.

Greenwalk, Howard P. *Organizations: Management without Control.* Thousand Oaks, CA: Sage Publications Incorporated, 2007.

Gross, C., P. Cary, Natalie Wong, Joel A. Dubin, Susan T. Mayne, and Harlan M. Krumholz. "Enrollment of Older Persons in Cancer Trials after the Medicare Reimbursement Policy Change." *Arch Intern Medicine* 165 (2005): 1514–20.

Health Care Financing Administration. "Protecting Your Health Insurance Coverage." 52, 2000.

History Makers, Medical Makers. "Dr. Harold Freeman Biography," http://www.thehistorymakers.com/biography/biography.asp?bioindex=109&category=medicalMakers.

History Makers, Medical Makers. "Lasalle Leffall," http://www.thehistorymakers.com/biography/biography.asp?bioindex=758.

Hogan & Hartson, LLP. "President Signs the Pediatric Research Equity Act of 2003 Requiring Specific Assessment of Safety and Efficacy in Children," 2003.

Honest Leadership and Open Government Act of 2007. 110-81. September 14, 2007.

Johnson, Randel K., and Katie Mahoney. "Re: Proposed Rule Regarding the Availability of Medicare Data for Performance Measurement." U.S. Chamber of Commerce, 2011.

Kaiser Family Foundation and National Women's Law Center. "Women's Access to Care: A State-Level Analysis of Key Health Policies," 2003.

Kalberer, Jr., John T. "Impact of the National Cancer Act on Grant Support." *Cancer Research* 35, (1975): 473–81, http://cancerres.aacrjournals.org/content/35/3/473.full.pdf.

Letter to the Subcommittee on Labor, Committee on Health and Human Services, Education, and Related Agencies, 2009.

Milligan, Chuck. "Reshaping Medicaid." National Governors Association.

National Institutes of Health. "Best Pharmaceuticals for Children Act (BPCA) Priority List of Needs in Pediatric Therapeutics." 17. Bethesda, MD: National Institutes of Health, 2011.

National Transitions of Care Performance & Metrics Work Group. "Improving on Transitions of Care: How to Implement and Evaluate a Plan." The National Transitions of Care Coalition, 2008.

Patient Protection and Affordable Care Act. 111-148. March 23, 2010.

The Pediatric Research Equity Act of 2003. 108-155.

Ranji, Usha, Alina Salganicoff, Alexandra M. Stewart, Marisa Cox, and Lauren Doamekpor. "State Medicaid Coverage of Perinatal Services: Summary of State Survey Findings." Kaiser Family Foundation and The George Washington University School of Public Health and Health Services, Washington, DC, 2009.

Rettig, Richard A. *Cancer Crusade: The Story of the National Cancer Act of 1971.* Princeton, NJ: Princeton University Press, 1977.

Smedley, Brian D. "Moving beyond Access: Achieving Equity in State Health Care Reform." *Health Affairs* 27, no. 2 (2008): 447–55.

Spulak, Thomas. "What's So Bad About Lobbyists, Anyway?" *The Hill* (2009). Published electronically January 13, 2009.

Unger, Joseph M., Charles A. Coltman Jr., John J. Crowley, Laura F. Hutchins, Silvana Martino, Robert B. Livingston, John S. Macdonald, Charles D. Blanke, David R. Gandara, E. David Crawford, and Kathy S. Albain. "Impact of the Year 2000 Medicare Policy Change on Older Patient Enrollment to Cancer Clinical Trials." *Journal of Clinical Oncology* 24, no. 1 (2006): 141–44.

U.S. Congress, 75th. National Cancer Act of 1937. Senate Bill 2067—Enacted August 5, 1937 (Public Law 244).

U.S. Congress. 79th. Hospital Survey and Construction Act (Hill-Burton Act). 1946.

U.S. Congress, 92nd. National Cancer Act of 1971. Senate Bill 1828—Enacted December 23, 1971 (Public Law 92-218).

U.S. Congress, 106th. Minority Health and Health Disparities Research and Education Act of 2000. Senate Bill 1880—Enacted October 31, 2000. (Public Law 106-525).

U.S. Congress, 107th. Best Pharmaceuticals for Children Act. Senate Bill 1789—Enacted January 4, 2002. (Public Law 107-109).

U.S. Department of Health and Human Services. *President Clinton Takes New Action to Encourage Participation in Clinical Trials: Medicare Will Reimburse for All Routine Patient Care Costs for Those in Clinical Trials*. Washington, DC: The White House Office of the Press Secretary, 2000.

Verdier, James, Margaret Colby, Debra Lipson, Samuel Simon, Christal Stone, Thomas Bell, Vivian Byrd, Mindy Lipson, and Victoria Pérez. "Soonercare 1115 Waiver Evaluation: Final Report." Washington, DC: Mathematica Policy Research, Inc, 2009.

Walsh, James. "Healthcare for Illegals Fits Leftist Goal of Plundering United States." *NewsMax,* October 12, 2009.

# CHAPTER 6

## Health Care Fraud

This chapter examines the idea that geographic variation in health disparities is, in part, explained by fraudulent conduct of health care delivery. In 2009, the federal government launched the Health Care Fraud Prevention and Enforcement Action Team (HEAT) program to combat fraud in Medicare. By the year 2010, HEAT had recovered more than two billion for the Medicare Trust Fund. Why did the government create HEAT? How does health care fraud influence the care of health disparity populations? How does the history of health care connect to our current understanding of fraud? Can policies designed to combat fraud change the pattern of health disparities in the United States? This chapter describes the history of health care delivery system financing that set the stage for the pervasiveness of fraud. It also examines the ACA's potential to decrease fraud. Ideally, a decrease in fraud will also decrease health disparities.

### PATIENT/SOCIETY VOICE

If you took the time to speak with a victim of health care fraud today, what would that victim say? Consider the experience of Norma Earl. All that Norma Earl originally wanted her home care nurse to do was take care of her cat. Earl said the woman soon started offering to pay her bills and clean her house while she was in the hospital, recovering from surgery. Investigators in the Utah Attorney General's Office said the nurse then started forging checks with Earl's name. "I got some of my bank statements," Earl recalled. "Some of my bills weren't being paid." When the damage was done, prosecutors said the nurse had taken more than 7,000 dollars from Earl who is a retired school teacher. The nurse was ultimately convicted and sentenced to probation. Earl finally received a check for the total restitution. The amount was 64 dollars and 90 cents. However, for Earl, it is bittersweet. "You just don't trust anybody," she told the Deseret Morning News.

What does fraud look or feel like from the perspective of a homeless person? The U.S. Attorney's Office speaks for these vulnerable individuals. The following is a press release from the U.S. Attorney's Office, Central District of California in Los Angeles, California. It was dated December 12, 2008. The press release describes what has become known as the *Skid Row* case:

## FORMER HOSPITAL CEO PLEADS GUILTY TO PAYING KICKBACKS IN "SKID ROW" HEALTH CARE FRAUD SCHEME

The former Chief Executive Officer (CEO) of City of Angels Medical Center pleaded guilty to paying illegal kickbacks for patient referrals in United States District Court in Los Angeles today. Rudra Sabaratnam, a sixty four year old physician from Brentwood, admitted to paying illegal kickbacks as part of a scheme to defraud Medicare and Medi-Cal by recruiting homeless persons from the Skid Row area of downtown Los Angeles.

Rudra Sabaratnam and his co-defendant, Estill Mitts also aged sixty four years old, of Los Angeles, are named in a twenty one count indictment that accuses both men of conspiring to recruit homeless people to receive unnecessary health services. Mitts pleaded guilty in September to conspiracy to commit health care fraud, money laundering, and tax evasion.

In pleading guilty, Sabaratnam admitted to paying Mitts and others to refer homeless Medicare and Medi-Cal beneficiaries whom they recruited, primarily from Skid Row, to City of Angeles for inpatient hospital stays. As part of the scheme, Sabaratnam entered into sham contracts intended to conceal the illegal kickbacks. Throughout the scheme, Mitts operated a facility called the Assessment Center, also known as Seventh Street Christian Day Center, located at 431 East Seventh Street, Los Angeles, California, in Skid Row. The total amount of illegal kickbacks that Sabaratnam paid and caused to be paid to Mitts and others was almost five hundred thousand dollars. City of Angels billed Medicare and Medi-Cal for inpatient services to the recruited homeless beneficiaries, including those for whom inpatient hospitalization was not medically necessary.

"This was a sophisticated scheme to defraud health care programs that are financed by taxpayers," said United States Attorney Thomas P. O'Brien. "These defendants stripped public health care programs of money that should have been used for those patients with legitimate needs, and are well deserving of prosecution by the United States."

The charges to which Sabaratnam has pleaded guilty carry a statutory maximum penalty of ten years in federal prison. Sabaratnam has agreed to pay over four million dollars in restitution to Medicare and Medi-Cal. United States District Judge George H. King ordered Sabaratnam to appear for sentencing on June 8, 2009.

The case against Sabaratnam and Mitts is part of an ongoing investigation being conducted by the United States Department of Health and Human Services, Office of the Inspector General; the Federal Bureau of Investigation; Internal Revenue Service, Criminal Investigation Division; the California Department of Justice Bureau of Medi-Cal Fraud and Elder Abuse; and the Health Authority Law Enforcement Team (HALT). This is a multi-agency task force which is operated by the Los Angeles County Department of Public Health.

Dr. Sabaratnam was actually sentenced to two years in prison and ordered to pay more than million dollars in restitution to the Medicare Trust Fund. This press release highlights the funds lost by Medicare and Medi-Cal. The U.S. Attorney's Office successfully completed this investigation by collaborating with the Health and Human Services. The homeless persons caught up in the scheme perpetrated by Sabaratnam and Mitts did not receive effective, preference-sensitive care. The government strike force was able to stop the crime, recover some funds, and identify an emerging scheme. Were the medically inappropriate treatments harmful for the individual victims? What became of these persons and their unmet medical needs? Skid Row is a neighborhood with other markers of health disparities—low income, limited literacy, and limited access to care. There are neighborhoods just like Skid Row scattered across the United States. This case illustrates the contribution that location makes to one's probability of encountering a fraudulent delivery system.

Can we find historical evidence of linking fraud with health disparities? One place to look is the history surrounding contaminated medicines and their detrimental impact on both the health and trust of African Americans. The Hampton Institute, an historically black college, issued a report in 1917, documenting the connection between illness and contaminated medicines:

> the credulity of the Negro has been capitalized, particularly in the South, by manufacturers of patent medicines according to a bulletin issued by Hampton Institute [in Norfolk, Virginia]. More than sixty percent of Negroes are addicted to the use of nostrums and in some districts of the South, one hundred percent. Large numbers of these false remedies cultivates the use of alcoholic liquors. Judging from advertising which is observable in many religious papers throughout the South, the Negro is not the only patent medicine guzzler in that region.

Patent medicine is a term associated with drug compounds in the 18th and 19th centuries in the United States. Often high in alcoholic content, these remedies were very popular with those who found this ingredient to be therapeutic. Many concoctions were fortified with morphine, opium, or cocaine. From the beginning, some physicians and medical societies were critical of patent medicines. They argued that the remedies did not cure illnesses, discouraged the sick from seeking legitimate treatments, and caused alcohol and drug dependency. By the end of the 19th century, Americans favored laws to force manufacturers to disclose the remedies' ingredients and use realistic language in advertising. In 1906, President Theodore Roosevelt signed the Pure Food and Drug Act, which led to action against unlabeled or unsafe ingredients, misleading advertising, the practice of quackery, and similar rackets. Patent medicines also led to mistrust of formal medical care. During a meeting of the North Atlantic Tuberculosis Conference in 1920, Major Allen Washington clearly links patent medicine with mistrust and delayed treatment for tuberculosis among African Americans in Virginia:

> It is estimated that in the State of Virginia . . . there are two thousand cases of tuberculosis among Negroes. It is our duty to see that this large percentage is lowered. One of the great troubles with our people in sickness is that many times they do not believe in a cure . . . the treatment is so simple that they have little faith in it. . . .

they often feel that the first thing to do is to go to a country store or to a quack doctor and purchase a patent medicine.

It has been true in many cases that when patients are suffering with tuberculosis they feel that they have been tricked by some enemy, and that the Conjure Doctor is the only person to help them. I have personally known of cases where whole families have been wiped out because of the failure to call in a real physician before the tubercular patient became too ill to be helped.

Fraud in health care delivery is not unique to the present. History shows us that fraud leads to mistrust, poor health, and premature death. The early 1900s were marked by a period of public health activism in the United States. There was advocacy for improved care for childbearing women and improved monitoring of the health of racial and ethnic groups. The National Center for Health Statistics did not track race and ethnicity statistics until the 1970s. Individuals were counted as white or nonwhite. There are scattered reports from large urban health departments about the mortality experience of African Americans and immigrants. Mothers dying in childbirth are the best measure of health from the early 1900s. In 1945, 20 of every 10,000 pregnant women died in childbirth. By 1965, the U.S. maternal death rate dropped by a factor of 10 to less than 3 per 10,000 persons. The drop in maternal deaths led to an increase in life expectancy to more than 70 years. Access to prenatal care and standardized obstetrical practices played a role. Indeed, the differences between black and white infant mortality rates converged for a while after 1965. There is clear evidence that this convergence is largely due to increased access to hospital care. There was also a boost in hospital revenues because Medicare financial incentives encouraged desegregation of hospitals.

Prior to the enactment of Medicare, personal finances limited access to hospital treatment. Older adults had the highest rates of poverty and were the group least likely to be admitted for treatment. During the late 1960s, Medicare financing led to gradual improvements in access to health care services by the elderly, the poor, and people of color. Medicare funds brought health care into geographic areas that were historically neglected. Before Medicare, rural areas were least likely to have a hospital. With the advent of payment, critical access hospitals (CAH) in rural areas became financially viable locations. Medicare improved access for a broad age range. In addition to serving the needs of older adults, CAHs provide maternity and pediatric care. With financial incentives, Medicare payment led to adoption of standardized treatments. These standards ensure that treatment is based on scientific evidence.

The impact of Medicare funding extends beyond direct payment for health care. Medicare payment now finances most segments of U.S. health care—institutional care, physician training—as well as providing investments in research infrastructure. All physicians are now required to train for a period of three to seven years after graduating from medical school. Through payments to these postgraduate training programs, Medicare supports the supply of all specialists—including pediatricians and obstetricians. The Association of American Medical Colleges provides oversight for these programs. Federal court rulings and civil rights activism forced desegregation of U.S. medical and nursing schools. Health care financing was instrumental in diversifying the health care workforce. Fueled by these new funds, the pharmaceutical, medical instrument, and supply industries rose to prominence on the New York Stock Exchange after 1965. Medical clinics also underwent great changes in function by the 1970s. Medicare was not the only factor influencing this historic improvement. Employer-sponsored insurance increased broad access to health care and is another factor financing access to health care. The *Stabilization Act* of 1942 (Public Law 77-729) had the unintended but positive effect of encouraging employer-sponsored health insurance as a benefit for U.S. workers. The changes resulting from the enactment of Medicare send a clear message that health disparities of all types— geographic, racial, and economic—can be improved with increased health care financing.

Payment policy plays a significant role by moving a health care system dominated by rigid financial segregation to one with open access to a broad range of groups. In the United States, health indicators for African Americans improved dramatically for a decade after 1965. The process of improved access began with the Hill Burton Hospital Construction Act of 1946. Hill Burton created financial incentives to replace an aging hospital infrastructure after the end of World War II. Was there fraud surrounding the implementation of Hill Burton? This is a question best left to medical historians. We can, however, ask a related question about the implementation of Medicare. Did this infusion of funds inadvertently contribute to the current pattern of health care fraud? Directly answering this question is a book-length analysis in its own right. Malcolm Sparrow at the Harvard Kennedy School of Government has written extensively on this issue. We can, however, improve our ability to see the connection. Local patterns of care provide clues.

Ultimately, all health care is local. Who is available in your neighborhood to provide care? How easy is it to be seen there? Since the enactment of Medicare, a transformation in health care delivery has taken place. The health care delivery experience has moved from a person whose office is down the street to a health care system with branches all over town. During the late 1950s and the early 1960s, the doctor's office was just around the corner from my grandmother's house. Good thing, too. I was accident prone. Not just little scrapes and bumps. No. At age three, I hit my head on the sharp edge of a piece of furniture. Off we went to the doctor's office. Dr. Dyer made it all better. No problem. At the end of the treatment, he warned my mom to watch me more closely. While playing on a wooden porch at age five, my leg went through a rotten floor board. The result was a nasty laceration consisting of a three-inch-long, two-inch-deep wound. Off we went to Dr. Dyer's office. At age seven, I fractured my wrist while playing. Again, Dr. Dyer saved the day. No getting in a car and driving to the hospital. No sitting in an emergency department for hours. Dr. Dyer knew me, my parents, and my siblings. He knew that these injuries were not child abuse. He knew I was a clumsy, adventuresome kid.

It is highly likely that Dr. Dyer trained at an historically black medical school. The choices in the 1950s were Howard University College of Medicine in Washington, DC or Meharry Medical College in Nashville, Tennessee. Howard's College of Medicine was signed into law by President Andrew Johnson on March 2, 1867, when Congress approved their charter to incorporate. Meharry was founded in 1876 as the Medical Department of Central Tennessee College in Nashville, under the auspices of the Freedman's Aid Society of the Methodist Episcopal Church. From the time of Howard's founding in the 1860s until the 1960s, Howard and Meharry trained almost all of the African American physicians in this nation. The core mission of each school was primary health care. Students were equipped to handle the challenges presented by a site that might not have all the technology that was needed. They were trained to overcome these deficiencies and deliver care to challenging patients. For most of the first half of the 20th century, many medical schools did not accept black students. Morehouse School of Medicine, another historically black college, did not open its doors until 1975. Dr. Dyer's office was located in an area of Kansas City, Kansas, known as the Northeast End. The Northeast End was a community whose residents' access to hospital care was limited. The local hospital—Douglas Hospital—was segregated. The Kansas University (KU) had a hospital that was approximately 10 miles from the Northeast part of town. In 1960, my family was reluctant to go there. That reluctance was based on their prior experience with the providers in those facilities. KU was better equipped. We did not, however, feel welcome. We did not trust the professionals who worked there to care about us. In the pre-Medicare era, segregated hospitals and care from a physician who lived in your community defined the delivery system for African Americans in a small Kansas town. Trust forged the link between provider and patient. Trust that the doctor had our best interests at heart and would give his or her best effort—despite limited technology. Trust that the cost of his or her care was determined through a fair process.

Currently, the U.S. health care system has grown to a business exceeding two trillion dollars per year. Fraud exploits the U.S. health care system that evolved after the implementation of Medicare. Our current legal approach to prosecuting fraud is guided by the False Claims Act 31 U.S.C. §§ 3729–33. The False Claims Act imposes liability on anyone who knowingly submits a false claim for payment to the U.S. Government. According to the Federal Bureau of Investigation (FBI), health care fraud costs the country an estimated 60 billion dollars a year. Fraud represents between 3 and 10 percent of Medicare expenditures in 2010. In addition to hurting our economy, legal scholar Joan Krause asserts that health care fraud hurts patients. Investigations by the U.S. Office of the Inspector General have identified a variety of schemes. Schemes used to perpetrate fraud include fake requests for payment, unnecessary medical procedures, ineffective lab tests, and utilization of goods and services under inappropriate circumstances. Funds recovered by successfully litigated FCA cases are distributed to the Medicare trust fund, federal agencies, and private parties who initiate civil suits on the government's behalf. These funds, however, are almost never distributed to the patients who may have been harmed by the fraudulent conduct. Indeed, the FCA does not provide redress for fraud-related injury for public plan beneficiaries. As has been pointed out by Krause, the *victim* is the federal bureaucracy. The goal of prosecution is returning funds to the federal treasury. Does the FCA diminish health disparities related to fraud? Is health care fraud so extensive that it makes a detectable contribution to population levels of physical illness, disability, and death?

The Robert Wood Johnson Foundation partnered with the Dartmouth Atlas Project to develop the Aligning Forces 4 Quality report. Their central observation is: "Who you are and where you live matters for volume *and quality* [author's italic] of health care received." Quality refers to the timing and appropriateness of care. This report explores the underlying causes of quality differentials within and across geographic regions. Fraud is not mentioned in any of the related reports from this collaboration. Rather, the authors identify unwarranted variations in health care. In their discussion, unwarranted refers to variation in medical practice or spending that cannot be explained by illness, strong scientific evidence, or well-informed patient preferences. Their data, derived from Medicare, acknowledges variation due to both *excessive* and *deficient* levels of service. In their view, appropriate care matches the population burden of illness. The Dartmouth Atlas Project describes three categories of appropriate care—effective care, preference-sensitive care, and supply-sensitive care. *Effective care* consists of evidence-based services. Variations in effective care often reflect failure to deliver service. This means that a necessary treatment is not received. *Preference-sensitive care* encompasses treatment decisions. The patient and the physician weigh options with different risks and benefits. Patient attitudes toward these risks may vary. At the end of the discussion, however, patient preferences lead to a decision about treatment. Failure to include individual preference can lead to over- as well as undertreatment. There are also issues surrounding *supply-sensitive care*. The number of hospital beds, the frequency of physician visits, and the tendency to consult a specialist are examples of supply-sensitive resources. The supply of these resources has a major influence on the likelihood of actual use. Excess supply has a clearly demonstrated link to excessive use. Excessive use means that the patient received a service where *none* is required. Since 2002, the Dartmouth Atlas Project has conducted analyses clearly showing the relationship between spending across geographic areas and differences in the quantity of supply-sensitive services. Regions differ dramatically in the use of the hospital. Hospital beds are a key indicator for supply-sensitive care. Areas with a large number of hospital beds tend to fill them. Blacks within a region are somewhat more likely than whites to be hospitalized for conditions that could also be treated outside of the hospital. Region is the most important determinant of utilization. Regional differences exceed the differences between racial groups living in the same region. Simply put, where you live determines the type and intensity of health care received. This simple observation underscores the importance of the local delivery system. These differences become clear when examining the following question. What is the predominant approach to selecting a site for care when a chronic disease needs treatment? Some local delivery systems emphasize acute, inpatient care while others emphasize ambulatory, outpatient care.

The Dartmouth analysis of claims data clearly show variation in Medicare spending across hospital regions. In Medicare data, hospital referral regions with the highest per capita cost are least likely to deliver preventive care. This means that a person 65 to 75 years of age with diabetes is less likely to have foot and eye examinations in areas with high hospital costs. Regular foot and eye examinations have been shown to decrease the risk of limb amputation and blindness among persons with diabetes. The Dartmouth Atlas Project rates of utilization for these preventive services are calculated using claims data. It is important that the reader understands that claims only measure payment. When fraudulent billing is a problem, actual care received cannot be accurately estimated from claims. Within the context of a discussion of fraud, this distinction is significant.

Paradoxically, patients in regions with high hospital costs report long waits for health care. High-cost regions have 32 percent more hospital beds, 31 percent more physicians, and 65 percent more specialists. Physicians in these areas are less likely to follow evidence-based guidelines for treatment of standard conditions. Facilities in these areas have little or no health information technology to support communication between sites of health care. In high-cost areas, there are higher mortality rates for diseases such as myocardial infarction, hip fracture, and colorectal cancer. In summary, anyone who receives care in a high-cost area is subject to the paradox of a large supply of hospital beds and specialists but longer waits for care. This paradox cuts across racial and ethnic groups. In high-cost areas, whites fare worse when compared to whites in low-cost areas. This suggests, but does not provide, evidence of fraud.

To fully illustrate the complex link in Medicare between high costs and poor outcomes for all patients, consider the data surrounding leg amputation. Amputation of a leg is an infrequent but devastating complication of peripheral vascular disease and diabetes. Environmental, behavioral, and social factors increase a person's risk for this complication of diabetes. Persons with low income and diabetes are more likely to have an amputation. Preventing amputation requires attention to foot care. Foot care includes daily examination and timely medical attention to calluses, blisters, or splinters. Prevention is a low-technology, low-profit activity. Among Medicare beneficiaries who have an amputation, more than 25 percent have a second amputation within a year and more than 30 percent die within the same period. Patients' risk for leg amputation varies depending on who they are and where they live.

Health disparities are defined by illness, disability, and mortality. Some areas of the United States have higher rates of disparities than others. Some areas perform less well on measures of health care quality. By comparing disparity rates, outcomes, and health care quality measures, we can look for the presence of health care fraud. Variation in quality, costs, and outcomes for racial groups in Medicare are well documented. In an age of international organized crime, incorporating measures of fraud into any study of health care inequity is necessary. By including fraud in our concept of health care inequity, evidence of mistrust of the health care system becomes a result of lived experience with service delivery—not an historical artifact related to a single government study of syphilis. Any business with a large economic impact has the potential to influence the patterns of health care. Health care is one-sixth of the U.S. economy. Health care, like every business, must contend with the problem of fraud within its ranks. The World Health Organization reports that almost 1 percent of the market value of medications in industrialized countries is counterfeit. IBM uses this fact to sell its process for tracking medication as it travels from the point of manufacturing to the patient's hand. Health disparities are a public health issue. According to the World Health Organization, counterfeit medications are also a public health issue. This is particularly true in countries where regulatory and enforcement systems for medicines are the weakest.

Is there a framework that could improve our ability to see fraud and its connection to disparities? In the mind of everyday citizens, health care fraud is viewed as white-collar crime involving commercial entities, doctors who submit false claims and other forms of dishonest business schemes. This perception has limitations. Public perception is not the only barrier to detecting health care fraud. According to law enforcement, it is difficult to build a credible legal case from a position outside of an organization. This problem is addressed by the False Claims Act. It encourages internal policing by permitting private citizens to sue on the government's behalf. These whistleblowers retain 15 to 30 percent of the proceeds obtained from a successful suit. Other barriers to detecting fraud stem from our roles as patient, provider, or payer. It is easier for payers to focus on wellness and prevention. Physicians are trained to believe in the quality of their tools. Patients are frightened by the idea that fraud may be involved in a life-threatening illness. These silos block our ability to take a broader view of the health care delivery system and detect fraud.

To develop the line of sight connecting fraud and disparity, let us use a metaphor about flight. The level of the flight can be (1) very high—50,000 feet, (2) somewhat high—5,000 feet, or (3) skimming across the ground at 5 feet. Fraud is both perpetrated and experienced at each of these levels. Developing a vertical view to see all levels is a challenge. The strategies used to perpetrate a scheme are different at each level. The experience of fraud is different at each level. The five-foot level of fraud looks a lot like street crime. It is a personal experience. It may or may not be perceived as fraud by the victim. Rather, the victim is embarrassed. The perpetrator is local. By contrast, 50,000 feet involves federal payment. Litigation at this level involves the FCA. These very different scenarios make discussions of fraud prevention and detection complicated. Antifraud advocates tend to focus on one level. While all advocates are passionate about the issue, there is a tendency to minimize the importance of elements that do not appear at one's own level and to maximize the importance of those that do. State agencies emphasize individual criminals operating locally—a five-foot view. Some advocates tend to view the issue as a problem with a singular hospital—a 5,000-foot view. Advocates of 50,000 feet emphasize corporate greed. The *Coalition against Insurance Fraud* (CAIF) is an example of this type of advocacy group. Formed in 1993, the CAIF is an alliance of insurance companies, consumer advocates, law enforcement, and civil rights groups. The National Urban League, a venerable civil rights organization, is a charter member but is more focused on loan fraud.

The health disparity discussion surrounding leg amputation and diabetes happens at a national level—50,000 feet. Medicare claims data, when viewed from the national level, clearly show racial disparities. The national average for amputation is 1 per 1,000 diabetic patients. Blacks were more likely to undergo amputation than whites—4 per 1,000 blacks compared to less than 1 per 1,000 whites. However, the variation in rates across regions of the United States is greater than the disparities between races within regions. Beneficiaries in McAllen, Texas, are 10 times more likely to have a leg amputation when compared to persons in Provo, Utah. Provo, Utah, has one of the lowest leg amputation rates in the United States. Wherever amputation rates are elevated for blacks, they are elevated for whites. In El Paso, Texas, the disparity between blacks and whites is similar—2 per 1,000 for blacks compare to slightly more than 1 per 1,000 for whites. In El Paso, Texas, the rate for each group is higher than the national average. In Oxford, Mississippi, amputation rates are among the highest in the nation. Blacks have a rate of more than 7 per 1,000 diabetic patients. The difference in amputation rates between white, diabetic Medicare patients living in Provo, Utah, and those living in Oxford, Mississippi, can be explained by health system factors. Again, these differences do not provide evidence of fraud. Fraud is just one of several potential explanations for regional variation in outcome. Leg amputation is a clinical procedure of last resort. It is used when treatment of a foot infection fails to respond to conservative measures. The process of amputation requires access to a surgical facility, skilled personnel, and medical equipment. Is the geographic variation in amputation explained, in part, by a bias toward profitable invasive medical practices?

In 2007, the Government Accounting Office (GAO) conducted a covert testing experiment to expose weaknesses in the procedures used to process the applications for vendors of *durable medical equipment*. The walkers and prosthetic limbs used by patients after surgery are a type of durable medical equipment. Investigators set up two fictitious companies using undercover names and bank accounts to create two durable medical equipment companies. The GAO designed the experiment to reflect practices used by criminals to fraudulently bill Medicare. The companies were approved for Medicare billing privileges despite having no clients and no inventory. The Centers for Medicare and Medicaid initially denied the GAO's application in part because of this lack of inventory. Undercover GAO investigators fabricated contracts with nonexistent wholesale suppliers to convince Centers for Medicare and Medicaid and its contractor, the National Supplier Clearinghouse (NSC), that the companies had access to durable medical equipment. The contact number the GAO gave for these phony contracts rang an unmanned undercover telephone in the GAO building. When NSC left a message looking for further information related to the contracts, a GAO investigator left a vague return message pretending to be the wholesale supplier. Simple methods of deception allowed the fictitious vendor and its wholesale supplier to obtain Medicare billing numbers. The weaknesses in the enrollment and inspection process allowed sham companies to fraudulently bill Medicare for unnecessary or nonexistent supplies. Real-world schemes like the GAO operation accounted for an estimate that Medicare improperly paid one billion dollars for durable medical equipment prosthetics and orthopedic supplies during the period of April 2006 through March 2007. The GAO experiment was structured to match the strategy used by a single company or a single delivery system at the 5,000-foot level.

Fraud is easier to detect in public plans. Reports about these plans provide clues that train our ability to see fraud at each level. Federal agencies are focused on the cost of fraud to public programs like Medicare and Medicaid. There is no formal consideration of individual injury. Public program enrollees are disproportionately older, female, and members of minority groups. Public program enrollees also tend to be less educated and have low incomes. Many of the ACA, Title VI polices specifically target Medicaid fraud. Medicaid is an easy target for fraudulent activity because it is a combination of vulnerable beneficiaries and administrative complexity. By virtue of their socioeconomic status, Medicaid recipients are our most vulnerable citizens—children, pregnant women, and the elderly, plus blind and disabled adults. Medicaid at the 50,000-foot level clearly has high cost and high utilization rates. The National Governors Association issued a white paper in 2010, emphasizing state budgetary stress created by the current demands on Medicaid. The analysis did not include an in-depth discussion of fraud.

The Skid Row case illustrates the connection between vulnerability and Medi-Cal from a 5,000-foot view. From a local level, there is competition between delivery systems. One makes excess profits—that is, Dr. Sabaratnam Assessment Center seemed to be a successful business model. Fraud is almost undetectable by individuals served by the center. Individuals felt as though they were getting attention that they had not been able to get before because many physicians refuse to see Medi-Cal patients. At the 5000-foot level are health care delivery systems—sites of care like hospitals, pharmacies, and regional long-term care facilities. Delivery systems range from aggregates of small, single offices to large, multisite corporate organizations. This broad range of systems reflects the fragmentation in U.S. health care. The Commonwealth Fund suggests that fragmentation contributes to its poor performance on quality measures such as preventive care and chronic care coordination. Fragmentation inhibits cross communication and increases the likelihood of fraud. Researchers link health disparities to a lack of accountability, a lack of care coordination, and difficulty accessing appropriate care. Fraud at this level is a *bad actor* type of crime. A single organization in a small region engages in fraudulent practices. Individual state Medicaid plans may disproportionately feel its impact when compared to Medicare. Medicaid-managed plans have only recently been evaluated for accountability, coordination, and ease of access by the National Committee on Quality Assurance since 2006. The report does not speculate about the potential for fraud to create these problems. However, there is clear variation in consumer ratings among these plans for ease of access to care. Fraud may be a barrier to achieving a high-performance health care delivery system. Delivery system fragmentation, particularly for Medicaid, creates an environment where fraud can flourish.

Fraud is most frightening when one is forced to think about being a victim. The emotional response of all crime victims involves a combination of fear, shame, and anger. Fear exists because fraud hurts. Whether justified or not, there is a sense of shame and personal responsibility. The desire for justice is fueled by anger. At the individual level, the experience of fraud is couched in emotional terms. Fraud victims are undetectable if they do not label themselves as victims. Observers can misattribute the emotional language of these victims to other factors. In research circles, delayed health care–seeking behaviors are attributed to mistrust of the system. In these conversations, mistrust is never linked to personal experience. Krause has collected testimonies from health care fraud victims. Their injuries fall into three categories of harm—financial, physical, and intangible. Excessive charges for medications requiring copayments have the potential to connect fraud with individual harm. Under Medicare Part B, beneficiaries are responsible for 20 percent of the cost of some outpatient cancer treatments. The cost of these medications can run into thousands of dollars. In 2001, Taketa Abbott Pharmaceutical Products, Inc. paid 875 million dollars to settle allegations of price inflation for the drug Lupron. Did individual patients get their excess co-payment dollars returned?

The complexity of the U.S. health care delivery system creates opportunity for fraud. At every point in the system, funds can be misdirected, starting with patients, employers, and taxpayers via government payouts. Each point of flow represents areas for potential fraud. Individuals pay directly out of pocket and in the workplace through benefit programs. In most cases, employers match the individual premiums and add more funds to the system. The government provides additional taxpayer money through its public programs. These programs include Medicare, Medicaid, the Veterans Health Administration, and the Indian Health Service. According to the Kaiser Family Foundation, more than two trillion dollars were spent on health care in 2008. Insurance programs—public and private—circulate this money through the system. As victims, consumers and insurance programs represent the highest and most lucrative targets for fraudulent activity. Insurance programs and providers can also be the target of fraudulent schemes at an intermediate level. This next level of fraud involves regional operators and limited types of services. Insurance programs are probably more aware of this fraud than individual providers. In addition to being victims, providers are also perpetrators of fraud. These *bad actors* make local headlines, and patients are victimized directly. Other members of the provider community are victimized by the mistrust that bad actors create.

Although these vulnerabilities extend to public and private plans alike, ACA Title VI focuses its fraud-control action on public plans. Public plans have more success obtaining court-based remedies. According to researchers and law enforcement agencies, this success is due to that fact that Medicare has an integrated database. There are a large number of patients in both programs. Medicare covers patients in all 50 states. Employers supporting employee insurance also experience increased costs associated with fraud. They would like to recover the money spent on these claims. A private plan would need to mine data from *all* the individual insurance plans offered to their employees to build a credible court case. These datasets are small and limited to specific employee groups. This data silo between employee health plans makes it difficult to accumulate sufficient evidence for legal action.

In addition to data silos, other practices increase the likelihood of successful fraud in the U.S. health care system. These practices include a fee structure that assumes veracity of claims, an automated claims-processing system dedicated to rapid payment, and a pay-and-chase approach to auditing claims. Ideally, these practices are designed to facilitate rapid payment. If the claims satisfy the criteria built into the system, they are assumed correct and are automatically paid. When there is a mistake, the assumption is that it is an error, not fraud. The default approach to any irregularity is to accommodate an honest but possibly overworked and error-prone physician. This default no longer reflects the current environment where the development of the codes for billing is a profit center for the American Medical Association. There is also a multimillion dollar business for training persons to translate an episode of care into a medical bill. Medical billing is promoted as a career track to administration. It is a common offering by proprietary schools. The pool of trained medical coders makes it simpler for an overworked and error-prone physician to contract out the claims preparation process.

Physical injury can happen as either an unintended consequence or as a direct result of unnecessary medical procedures. For example, prosecutors settled allegations that cardiac surgeons at Shasta Regional Medical Center (SRMC), formerly known as Redding Medical Center, performed unnecessary heart surgeries on as many as 700 patients. These procedures included open heart and coronary bypass surgeries. Most of these patients lived in the area surrounding SRMC. How many developed complications that led to new diseases, new disabilities, or death? An example of intangible harm includes fraudulent use of health care information to obtain reimbursement for services not performed. What happens to your ability to purchase new insurance if your medical records falsely contain a chronic condition? In each of these three instances—financial, physical, or intangible—individual patients are harmed. Are their injuries routinely addressed through the formal legal process? No. It is possible that sufficient numbers of victims are concentrated in a small enough geographic area to alter public health measures of death, illness, and injury. Credible estimates from public health departments are needed to confirm this view.

Medicare's pay-and-chase approach to auditing a small sample of claims after payment is a process called post-payment utilization review. At all levels, successful fraud is possible when the perpetrator carefully crafts the bogus claim. Without the patient's knowledge, an entire episode of care can be fabricated. The audit is focused on medical appropriateness, not the verification of the actual service. Fraud perpetrators fabricate records, using the U.S. Preventive Services Task Force guidelines to create fictitious claims. Prevailing audit practices at the utilization review involve mailing requests for copies of the relevant medical record to providers. To pass these audits, fraud perpetrators consistently lie twice. The FBI has identified fraud in a variety of forms—fraudulent billings, medically unnecessary services or prescriptions, kickbacks, and duplicate claims are a few. These schemes target individual health care beneficiaries as well as large health care programs like Medicare and Medicaid. Perpetrators are found across a spectrum including vendors, medical facilities and laboratories, suppliers of medical equipment, organized crime groups, corporations, and sometimes the beneficiaries themselves. Fraud is associated with organized crime, gangs, and cybercrime.

ACA Title VI, Transparency and Program Integrity, is designed to correct characteristics that create points of vulnerability. These provisions target fraudulent data schemes and predatory business practices as well as creating new legal tools and penalties. Step one involves dismantling the data silos (Sections 6503, 6504, 6507, 6603, 6606, and 6607). Another step involves refining business practices that have been employed in other fraud cases. These practices include defining allowable business affiliations under Medicaid (Section 6502), stopping Medicaid payments to organizations outside of the United States (Section 6505), allowing states to correct federal determinations of overpayment using the new Medicaid Management Information System (Section 6506), and prosecuting false marketing claims made by health insurance plans (Section 6601). These policies extend protections to private health insurance markets including individual, small group, and large group plans. There are also new legal tools available for states (Section 6604) and employer-sponsored plans (Section 6605). Section 6604 allows the federal government to apply state fraud statutes to cases where federal law is otherwise silent. Section 6605 gives the U.S. Department of Labor the authority to issue Cease and Desist Orders for financially unstable health plans. Prior to the enactment of this section, the government had no recourse to protect insurance purchasers from financially unstable insurers. Finally, the ACA has created new penalties for perpetrators. Formerly, a business engaging in fraud could be barred from future participation in Medicare. However, there was no communication between Medicare and Medicaid. At present, there is bidirectional notification for Medicare (federal) and Medicaid (state) when a business is barred under Medicare or any other state plan. This penalty is designed to stop fraudulent businesses from moving to a new location to renew their fraudulent practices (Section 6501).

The Medicare Fraud Strike Force (MFSF) was launched in 2007. The collaboration brings together the U.S. Attorney's Office with the HHS. The MFSF was created to handle chronic fraud and emerging schemes. Its stated goal is prosecuting individuals and entities that do not provide legitimate health care services and who exist for the sole purpose of defrauding government health care programs. To date, the schemes are broad in scope. Some consist of fraudulent claims to Medicare for durable medical equipment—power wheelchairs and orthotics, compound medications for use in therapies, HIV infusion clinics, tube feeding, and fraudulent billing companies. These services are not inherently fraudulent. Individuals with a variety of illnesses derive benefit from wheelchairs, outpatient treatments, and tube-feeding. Unfortunately, some companies use this need to obtain extra payments. Prosecutors are now expanding their investigation of targeted schemes to include home health agencies and independent diagnostic testing facilities.

## SUMMARY AND IMPLICATIONS

This chapter explores the connection between health disparities and health care fraud. Is there historical evidence that fraud can cause disparities? Yes. Is there current data that fraud contributes to geographic variation in U.S. health care quality? Not yet. This chapter is not designed to lay blame on any single health care sector for fraudulent practices. Rather, by forging a link between health disparities and fraud, the work of health equity advocates can be enhanced. Both patients and providers—physicians, nurses, and other workers—are victimized by fraud. Naiveté limits the ability of good people to put the pieces together. Fear, apathy, and mistrust blind patients to the possibility of fraud. A fearless, clear-eyed review of the facts is required for resolution of these issues. Health disparities are not uniformly distributed across the United States. There is geographic variation in the size and composition of health disparities. Murray and colleagues (2006) describe this as the "Eight Americas." Eight separate Americas can be defined by a combination of race, county of residence, and death rates. The geographic differences in death rates are not completely explained by socio-demographic factors like income. The authors describe variation using the following language:

> Disparities in mortality cross the eight Americas, each consisting of millions or tens of millions of Americans, are enormous by all international standards. The observed disparities in life expectancy cannot be explained by race, income, or basic health-care access and utilization alone. Because policies aimed at reducing fundamental socioeconomic inequalities are currently, practically absent in the United States, health disparities will have to be at least partly addressed through public health strategies that reduce risk factors for chronic diseases and injuries.

The ACA contains antifraud provisions that have the potential to decrease health disparities. Title VI is based on government's experience with successfully litigated fraud cases. Some cases are linked to services not delivered. Other cases link fraud to substandard medication and equipment. By improving transparency in the payment process, we will improve our ability to see these linkages. The inclusion of fraud in the list of health disparity factors requires cognitive rather than legislative process. Sometimes it is difficult to find an object right in front of your face until you say its name out loud. The link between health disparities and fraud may operate in a similar fashion. After reading this chapter, some readers will remain skeptical that fraud could make a substantial contribution to health disparities. Trust is a component of health care. Disturbing that trust has considerable consequences for persons on both sides of the stethoscope. Trust, however, can be strengthened when the patient and the provider communicate about all aspects of treatment. If a patient does not improve, then a provider must entertain the possibility of substandard medication. Sometimes individuals with the best of intentions are most vulnerable to fraud. If the government was not involved in financing care, would health disparities persist? In her testimony to the U.S. Senate Committee on Health Education Labor and Pensions, Dr. Alieta Eck argued that free clinics are sufficient to address the needs of the poor (May 11, 2011): "In the United States, people aren't dying in the streets."

As a final thought, let us examine the current environment of charity clinics. These are clinics where government intervention is minimized or eliminated altogether. What if the City of Angels Clinic, operated by Dr. Sabaratnam, had been a charity clinic with sole support from philanthropic funds and staffed by volunteers? Clearly, Medicare/Medi-Cal fraud would not be possible. Would the center's patients still be vulnerable to fraud-induced injury? Yes. By not accepting public insurance plans like Medicare or Medicaid, free clinics are not subject to payment policies designed to promote quality in health care. The ACA contains a policy extending medical malpractice coverage to personnel working at free clinics. Why malpractice coverage specifically for free clinics? Extending malpractice coverage is designed to support the financing of these facilities and attract frontline professionals to serve. What does a well-run charity clinic look like? Consider the Rhode Island Free Clinic:

"The Free Clinic, based in Providence, offers primary care to uninsured adults who earn less than one hundred fifty percent of the federal poverty level which comes to more than twenty seven thousand per year for a family of three. The clinic accepts no government or insurance money, relying entirely on donations and volunteer labor to handle about two thousand visits a year. Everyone is keenly aware of what it means to be laid off," says Julie White, the clinic's director of development. "That means you're no longer insured. The uninsured are in every community across the state."

(Pro7 to 7, February 2009)

This facility is staffed by volunteer health care workers. Will their patients be less likely to suffer from health disparities? If a reduction in health disparities is linked to a consistent flow of appropriate medication, then the answer is "No." The Rhode Island Free Clinic's new pharmacy service has 50 common generic drugs that are freely given away to clinic patients. The ability to provide medications at no charge has caused a lot of excitement among clinic doctors:

"This was a huge landmark for us, a real breakthrough in our mission. You can't talk about primary care without providing the pharmaceuticals. Otherwise it's just diagnosis, not treatment" says White. "Now we know we are completing the circle."

Purchased with money raised from foundations, the drugs in the pharmacy are available only to clinic patients with a prescription from a clinic doctor. The pharmacy stocks medications for the most common conditions: high blood pressure, high cholesterol, back pain, depression, or diabetes. Patients who need a branded drug or a drug not in the formulary are connected to drug makers' assistance programs for the poor or supplied with free samples. Clinic patients are selected in a monthly lottery—a process the clinic hopes to eliminate but still needs because it cannot meet the demand. For these persons—many of whom are young and middle-aged adults without health insurance—inability to obtain consistent health care is an inequity. Unemployed persons relying on a lottery system to obtain chronic medications for high blood pressure, depression, or diabetes is an inequity. Free clinics have the unintended potential to mask the full extent of health care disparities. Ultimately, patients are unable to distinguish between reputable operations like the Rhode Island Free Clinic and places like City of Angels. Free clinics do not hold much promise to decrease health disparities. Their vulnerability to health care fraud is just one among many reasons.

Fraud in the delivery of health care is a reality. It is most likely to happen when criminals see an opportunity—that is, a vulnerable population. There are legal tools available to patients who are victims of fraud. The common legal view of fraud in the United States rests primarily on violations of health care payment policies. When a health care delivery entity operates outside of public payment rules, the protection available to providers and patients are less clear. Persons who are forced to seek care outside of these protections are the most vulnerable to fraud. Clinics that support their activities through philanthropy operate outside of the payment policy framework established by Medicare and Medicaid as well as the Employer Retirement Income Security Act of 1974 (ERISA). Each of these programs has extensive rules designed to protect the interests of patients. These rules include policies concerning provider screening and enrollment requirements and standards for evidence-based management of disease. When an FCA settlement is won, there are no defined remedies for patients in free clinics. In short, free clinics are markers of inequity. These clinics do not resolve underlying care access issues nor do they protect patients from fraud-related injury. A potential unintended consequence is that they may create an environment that allows fraud to flourish. ACA Title I, II, and VI begin the process of moving these facilities toward higher standards of care while protecting both providers and patients. As long as the United States has economic apartheid in health care, it will have conditions that encourage fraud.

## BIBLIOGRAPHY

*Advocate* 3, no. 44 (1917), http://www.infoweb.newsbank.com.

Almond, Douglas V., Kenneth Y. Chay, and Michael Greenstone. "The Civil Rights Act of 1964: Hospital Desegregation and Black Infant Mortality in Mississippi." NBER Working Paper JEL No. J15, I18, I11, I38, N32, 2008, 38.

Federal Bureau of Investigation. "Health Care Fraud: Trends and Tips," http://www.fbi.gov/news/stories/2010/june/health-care-fraud/health-care-trends.

Fisher, Elliott S., David C. Goodman, and Amitabh Chandra. "Regional and Racial Variation in Health Care among Medicare Beneficiaries: A Brief Report of the Dartmouth Atlas Project." In *Aligning Forces for Quality: Improving Health and Health Care in Communities across America*, edited by Kristen K. Bronner. Princeton, NJ: Robert Wood Johnson Foundation, 2008.

Goodarz, Danaei, Eric B. Rimm, Shefali Oza, Sandeep C. Kulkarni, Christopher J. L. Murray, and Majid Ezzati. "The Promise of Prevention: The Effects of Preventable Risk Factors on National Life Expectancy and Life Expectancy Disparities by Race and County in the United States." *PLoS Medicine* 7, no. 3 (2010): e1000248.

Goodman, David C., and Elliott S. Fisher. "Physician Workforce Crisis? Wrong Diagnosis, Wrong Prescription." *New England Journal of Medicine* 358 (2008): 1685–61, http://www.nejm.org/doi/full/10.1056/NEJMp0800319.

Government Accountability Office. "Gao-08-955—Medicare: Covert Testing Exposes Weaknesses in the Durable Medical Equipment Supplier Screening Process." GAO Reports and Comptroller General Decisions, Washington, DC, 2008.

Hetzel, Alice M. "History and Organization of the Vital Statistics System." National Center for Health Statistics, 1997.

"History of the Pure Food and Drug Act." http://www.hagley.lib.de.us/library/exhibits/patentmed/history.

Jinkook, Lee, and Horacio Soberon-Ferrer. "Consumer Vulnerability to Fraud: Influencing Factors." *Journal of Consumer Affairs* 31, no. 1 (1997): 70–89, http://www.eric.ed.gov/ERICWebPortal/search/detailmini.jsp?_nfpb=true&_&ERICExtSearch_SearchValue_0=EJ542232&ERICExtSearch_SearchType_0=no&accno=EJ542232.

Jones, James H. *Bad Blood: The Tuskegee Syphilis Experiment*. New York: The Free Press, 1993.

Kavilanz, Parija. "Health Care: A 'Goldmine' for Fraudsters." *CNNMoney.com,* 2010. Published electronically January 13, 2010. http://money.cnn.com/2010/01/13/news/economy/health_care_fraud/.

Kimbuende, Eric, Usha Ranji, Janet Lundy, and Alina Salganicoff. "United States Health Care Costs, Background Brief." Kaiser Family Foundation, Washington, DC, 2010.

Krause, Joan H. "Promises to Keep: Health Care Providers and the Civil False Claims Act." *Cardozo Law Review* 23 (2002): 1363–418.

Miles, Toni P. "Impact of Reform in the United States Health Care Markets on Health Disparities." *Public Policy and Aging Report* 19, no. 4 (2010): 15–18.

Mrozek, Thom. "Former Hospital CEO Pleads Guilty to Paying Kickbacks in 'Skid Row' Healthcare Fraud Scheme." Department of Justice, 2008.

Murray, Christopher J. L., Sandeep C. Kulkarni, Catherine Michaud, Niels Tomijima, Maria T. Bulzacchelli, Terrell J. Landiorio, and Majid Ezzati. "Eight Americas: Investigating Mortality Disparities across Races, Counties, and Race-Counties in the United States." *PLoS Medicine* 3, no. 9 (2006): e260. Published electronically September 12, 2006, http://www.plosmedicine. org/article/info:doi/10.1371/journal.pmed.0030260.

National Committee for Quality Assurance. "Health Plan Report Card," http:// reportcard.ncqa.org/plan/external/.

Pro7 to 7. February 2009, http://news.providencejournal.com/breaking-news/ 2009/02/ri-free-clinic.html#.T1zX1Hmgx3E.

Rosenbaum, Sara, Nancy Lopez, and Scott Stifler. "Health Insurance Fraud: An Overview." Robert Wood Johnson Foundation, 2009.

Scott, George. "Stronger Department of Education Oversight Needed to Help Ensure Only Eligible Students Receive Federal Student Aid. Report to the Chairman, Subcommittee on Higher Education, Lifelong Learning, and Competitiveness, Committee on Education and Labor, House of Representatives." U.S. Government Accountability Office, 2009.

Sparrow, Malcolm K. "Fraud in the United States Health Care System: Exposing the Vulnerabilities of Automated Payment Systems." *Social Research* 75, no. 4 (2008).

U.S. Congress, 77th. The Stabilization Act of 1942. Public Law 77-729, 56 Stat. 765. Enacted October 2, 1942.

U.S. Congress, 79th. Hospital Survey and Construction Act of 1946. Public Law 725, Code 42, Session 79.

*Washington Bee.* October 23, 1920, http://www.infoweb.newsbank.com.

Winslow, Ben. "Fraud Victims Speak out on White Collar Crime." *Deseret Morning News.* Published electronically November 1, 2007, http://www. allbusiness.com/crime-law-enforcement-corrections/criminal-offenses- fraud/14454622-1.html.

# CHAPTER 7

## Young Adults

On March 15, 2011, the following obituary was published in a small Midwestern newspaper:

> Born December 19, 1985, Miss Georgia Jones joined her heavenly father. She is survived by her mother and father, two sisters, two brothers, her grandparents, and host of aunts, uncles, cousins, nephews, and other relatives who loved her very much.

Georgia was chronologically only 25 years old, but after years of struggle with cerebral palsy, her body was biologically similar to that of a woman in her 80s. Her survival was largely attributable to the care she received from her family. Their caregiving was supplemented by resources purchased with state Medicaid funds. Her story began in 1984, when the steel mill that employed her father went out of business. He was 32 years old at the time. His young wife was pregnant with Georgia. The loss of this job meant a loss of health care insurance without other options for obtaining other coverage. Consolidated Omnibus Budget Reconciliation Act (COBRA) did not become law until 1986. Today, COBRA offers unemployed workers the opportunity to maintain health insurance if the worker can continue to pay the premiums for membership in the group policy. COBRA was not enacted soon enough to prevent the loss of health care experienced by Georgia's mom. The loss of health care and subsequent complications led to Georgia's cerebral palsy. Her story carries three lessons. First, there are critical periods in the life of a child when health care cannot wait. Second, Medicaid is the only lifeline of support for families with disabled children. Finally, as children with disabilities reach adulthood, the access to health care becomes increasingly tenuous. In Georgia's case, she needed home-based services to supplement the caregiving provided by her family. Some of the costs of these services were offset by Medicaid. When her father found a new job, Georgia was ineligible for his new employer-sponsored insurance. Throughout her short 25-year life, Georgia and her parents encountered multiple and unexpected barriers to obtaining health care. This chapter describes the experiences of young adults as they navigate the health care landscape. Young adult life is marked by transitions. As we shall see in this chapter, unanticipated barriers emerge during these transitions. Does the ACA resolve the barriers that are unique to young adult life?

Transitions are the trickiest part of life. Young adults are moving from dependence on parental resources to independence. Independently accessing basic health care is a very complex transition in the United States. To develop an accurate picture of the health care system encountered by young adults, we need to hear what they have to say. While the opinions of Medicare beneficiaries appeared in news reports every day during the health reform debate, the voices and experiences of young adults were less well represented. Organizations like the Commonwealth Fund conducted surveys of young adults to fill this void. Are their requests reflected in the final version of the ACA? In 2009, the Commonwealth Fund conducted a survey of adults aged 19 to 29. They found that 98 percent of Democrats, 88 percent of Independents, and 73 percent of Republicans felt it was important to pass some type of health care reform legislation. Sixty-two percent of survey participants supported the idea of individual responsibility for purchasing one's own health insurance. In this group, 44 percent reported having health insurance coverage through an employer-sponsored plan—their own or from parents. These opinions were formed in a health care environment not designed to explicitly support the transition that every young adult makes from being a dependent to being an independent person. Almost half of the 20 million adults in this age group were uninsured during 2009. Most of these have been uninsured for two or more years. Health care access inequities are a fact of life for adults aged 19–29.

There are other examples of advocacy for young adults during construction of the ACA. Howard Dean summarizes the cost-based rationale in an interview for *Time* magazine:

*Time* magazine: In your book, you talk about how someone's age deter-mines his attitude toward having health insurance. You say the federal gov-ernment should provide free coverage to everyone under age thirty. That's radical.

Dean: It's incredibly cheap. Statistically, only two expensive things hap-pen to people under age thirty years. One is malignancy, and the other is an accident. Everything else is mostly preventive maintenance and it's very inexpensive.

Dr. Dean is correct that the overall cost to government and society to provide health care for this group is cheap when compared to other age groups. He uses this cost to society-based rationale for promoting univer-sal health insurance to cover young adults and their families. This view, however, misses the burden that illness creates for individuals. This chap-ter combines stories and statistics to fully describe the circumstances of individual young adults who require health care. Are there solutions to these problems in the ACA? Why a specific focus on young adults? More than 50 years of research demonstrates that adult transitions— independence, family formation, and entry into the workforce—are ex-periences associated with prolonged absence of health care access. The ACA contains policies that recognize these gaps. These policies include individual and employer responsibility, essential benefits, the Medicaid expansion, and some demonstration projects involving long-term care. Each has the potential to prevent the scenario that defined Georgia's life.

The first critical transition all teenagers make is the transition from dependence to independence. In the United States, this begins with high school graduation. The transition is so treacherous for high school drop-outs that their experiences are not covered in this chapter. The Anne E. Casey Foundation has published several comprehensive reports en-titled *Kids Count* on this issue. It is a detailed discussion of these young adults. Rather, this discussion is limited to the usual or more common pattern of transition. High school graduation is a critical period for all kids covered by parental health insurance. Before the ACA, almost all employer-sponsored plans ended coverage at age 19. Some plans ex-tended coverage an additional four years for students going to college. High school graduates who did not go straight to college were faced with three scenarios: go without health insurance, apply for Medicaid, or obtain employer-sponsored coverage. It is important to recognize that unemployment does not make one eligible for Medicaid. Recent high school graduates do not have the COBRA option. The net effect of graduation without the prospect of employment means going without health insurance for most kids.

Disability is one criterion that might qualify a new high school graduate for Medicaid. This was Georgia's transition to adulthood. She graduated from high school with a combination of home and public school support. Society has become increasingly aware of kids with disabilities. A series of court cases and advocacy culminated in the Americans with Disabilities Act (1990) and the Olmstead Amendment (2008). These landmark laws have increased the access of young adults to mainstream society over the past 20 years. Americans with disabilities make a significant contribution to the U.S. gross domestic product through their participation in the workforce. In 2010, more than 28 percent of persons with disabilities were employed. Young adults with disabilities are most sensitive to changes in employer-sponsored insurance costs, benefit changes, and barriers related to preexisting conditions. While Medicaid is not an option for young adults with jobs, many find that their employer-sponsored insurance does not provide the specialized equipment needed to fully integrate into society. Recent high school graduates are in a particularly vulnerable situation. Will they find a job that provides insurance? In 2009, 59 percent of all high school graduates found employment. In 2011, the Bureau of Labor Statistics reported that the median salary of a full-time worker aged 16 to 24 was 433 dollars per week. This salary places these workers in the bottom quarter of all wage earners. Whether they are unemployed or working in low-wage jobs, young adults fresh out of high school are up against a wall.

Dean's perception that this group is cheap to cover ends with the reality of out-of-pocket spending for health care among young adults. To show the dollars and cents associated with this problem, Geoffrey Paulin used the Consumer Expenditure data to examine health care spending by young adults and their families. He reports that in 2008, almost one million persons aged 18 to 24 paid for a visit to the emergency department. The annual costs for this visit ranged from almost 300 dollars to more than 5,000 dollars. During the same year, almost two million young adults purchased prescription medications. The annual costs for those medications ranged from 1,200 dollars to more than 72,000 dollars. Overall, more than three million young adults paid for some type of health care. Those costs ranged from more than 3,000 dollars to more than half a million dollars. These expenditures represent a year's worth of the out-of-pocket costs for accidents, pregnancy, chronic medications, and other health care needs.

In almost all cases, the expenses were managed with credit cards. Young adults—particularly those with disabilities—are missing from Dr. Dean's sound bite. More than 15 percent of young adults have some form of disability. Mental disorders are the number one cause of disability for this age group. Chronic mental illness usually appears in young adulthood. For example, the first episode of manic depression costs an average of one-half million dollars. These dollars go beyond health care to include legal fees, housing issues, and other expenses related to the sudden onset of manic behavior. If the transition from dependence on parental insurance is accompanied by limited education, joblessness, or disability, it is a starting place for the emergence of health disparity. Title I of the ACA extends parental coverage until the age of 26 for all kids—whether they attend college or not. Universal extension of health insurance coverage to age 26 could diminish the health care inequities associated with young adulthood. Kids in foster care with Medicaid coverage also received the age extension. Kids whose parents become unemployed during their transition do not have a place in this legislation.

The next critical transition for many young adults is the formation of a family. The formation process involves personal relationships, acquisition of skills for the job market, and timing of a pregnancy. As the reader knows, there is no orderly process for bringing these pieces together. For many young adults, these events often happen simultaneously. Consider this sentiment from a member of the University of Louisville Moms Club. This is a group of young women simultaneously raising kids and attending college:

> My husband and I are both working full time jobs and going to school. These jobs pay ten dollars per hour. Neither of us had health insurance—so buying the pill was not an option. We used rubbers but you know that sometimes they just fail. Anyway, when I went to apply for Passport [Kentucky Medicaid], they treated me like I was a slacker. I do not believe in abortion and we are going to school so that we can make more money. I was eligible and we got what we needed. I just hate being treated like I am doing something wrong.
>
> (Personal communication)

Health care is required for a mother and child to successfully complete a pregnancy. In 2009, almost 50 percent of all births were supported with Medicaid funds. This support was necessary because one-third of all births were to women aged 24 and younger. Whether married or not, this age group is most likely to be unemployed or working in low-wage jobs without insurance. During the 1960s and 1970s, when most boomer women had their children, maternity coverage was an essential feature of employer-sponsored health insurance. Hospital stays for a normal delivery ranged from three to five days. During that time, mothers could rest, recover, and receive training in infant care. In the 2000s, a childbearing woman is a member of Generation X (Gen X). These women have a very different experience. In order to obtain health insurance, Gen X women know that they must apply for Medicaid or purchase a maternity care plan in the private insurance markets. This plan may or may not include prenatal visits or treatment for complications associated with the pregnancy. Members of the University of Louisville Moms Club, like all Gen X women, expect to be discharged from the hospital in 24 to 48 hours. The new mother is instructed to bring the baby back to the doctor if the child is not doing well. Communication between the current cohort of childbearing women and boomer women is complicated. Policy makers who had the boomer experience of supported childbirth assume that Gen X women share the same experience. On the other hand, young adults do not know that access has changed. This is clearly an intergenerational difference in health care access. It has implications for the pattern of health disparities in the future. A Casey Foundation report described the experience of some 850,000 Gen X mothers who were under the age of 20 years. Fifty percent of these women no longer live with their parents, and many are head of their own household. The Casey Foundation advocates for young adults who are not always tuned into the details of public policy. These mothers, however, understand the day-to-day experience of unmet medical needs. Their unmet medical needs have the potential to become health disparities during the lifetime of their families.

To further illustrate the experience of today's young parents, consider Kathy's story. She is a 38-year-old single mother with two boys aged 20 and 16 years. Last year she earned 50,000 dollars in her job as an information technology specialist working for private medical practices in the Dallas-Fort Worth area. This position places her inside specialty medical practices across the area to hear the conversations of physicians involved in the ACA. She is a contract worker. Twenty years ago, she might have been employed by a company with group benefits. Today, she purchases private health insurance as a single person. She is faced with the following insurance choices: a family plan with 700 dollars per month in health insurance premiums and a 5,000 dollar deductible or a single plan for each child at 50 dollars per month—100 dollars total per month and the prospect of doing without health insurance for herself. At 50,000 dollars of pretax income, her yearly salary is just beyond the Texas Children's Health Insurance Program (CHIP) eligibility limit of 38,000 dollars for a family of three. If Texas CHIP provides insurance for each of her sons, the savings would allow Kathy to purchase a single policy to cover her own health care. Although Kathy's eligibility is calculated on pretax income, she pays for health care out of posttax, take-home wages of approximately 3,100 dollars per month. These wages must cover the average monthly rent of 900 dollars for a two-bedroom apartment in Dallas, the average monthly utility cost of 100 dollars, and an average daily commute of 50 miles round trip that costs 240 dollars per month for gas. After paying for these necessities, she has approximately 1,900 dollars for everything else. Her final decision was to purchase a policy covering the kids and pay for her own expenses using a Health Savings Account. Created in 2003 as part of the Medicare Prescription Drug, Improvement, and Modernization Act, a Health Savings Account is designed to allow consumers to direct their health care expenses. The basic package consists of a low-premium insurance policy, a high annual insurance deduction, and a tax-free savings account to use for medical expenses. The economic rationale for this choice is based on the savings achieved with lower insurance premiums and taxes. Analyses of the reality surrounding health savings accounts paint a slightly different picture. In a traditional employer-sponsored health insurance plan, the individual premium dollars are matched by employer dollars. These paired dollars are useful for purchasing plans with a larger menu of benefits and a lower annual deduction—usually 500 dollars or less. In contrast, employers do not match health savings accounts dollars. The annual deductible for these nontraditional plans averages 5,000 dollars per year. In Kathy's case, this deductible is 10 percent of her pretax income. Finally, the tax benefit associated with a health savings account is a deduction to taxes—not a tax credit. According to analyses by the U.S. Department of the Treasury, a family of four needs an income of 120,000 dollars and a contribution of 2,000 to their health savings account to get a tax savings of 620 dollars. What is the bottom line? The health savings account is most attractive to healthy individuals with few medical expenses. Persons with chronic conditions—like asthma or a disability—are more likely to reach the 5,000 dollar deductible each year. While the majority of young adults are healthy individuals with few medical expenses, more than 15 percent of adults aged between 18 and 24 have a disability. Does the ACA contain policies to alter the barriers experienced by these young adults as they transition from dependence to independence? Does this insurance package meet Kathy's needs? Kathy's experience with her injury clearly shows the limits of the health savings accounts strategy.

In February of 2010, Kathy fractured her lower leg in a fall on an icy sidewalk. The cost of her initial surgery in a day hospital amounted to 30,000 dollars. Her employer, an orthopedic surgeon, gave her a discount that included free physical therapy. Otherwise, each visit would cost 75 dollars. This procedure did not include 1,000 dollars for the cost of anesthesia; 500 dollars for the emergency room visit; 3,400 dollars for the emergency room physician; almost 700 dollars for the ambulance ride; and 300 dollars for the medical equipment—air boot, brace, and other items. Before the injury, her health savings account was depleted by the costs of eyeglasses and dental care purchased for her boys. Her comment on these medical bills:

I feel sorry for patients. My bill could have been more—I got a break.

Our interview took place in August. She is still paying off the tab one monthly payment at a time. Her surgery required placement of pins in the fractured leg. These pins need to be removed once healing has taken place. She was told that the pins need to be in place for at least one year. She is pushing her doctor to remove the pins early—waiting a complete year means that she will need to pay another annual deductible for the second surgery. What are the health care needs of young adults? Most need basic health insurance for maternity care, health coverage for their families, and coverage for accidental injury. They also need insurance that is afford-able to a wage earner at or below a median income of 40,000 dollars. Currently, the only change to health savings accounts that might affect Kathy is Section 9003, effective from December 2010. She will no longer be able to pay for nonprescription medications tax free using these funds. Before ACA, purchasers always paired health savings accounts with high-deductible, limited-benefit insurance plans. High-deductible plans also exclude medical care for pregnancy and preventive services as an addi-tional strategy to keep costs low. Finally, cost control is also achieved by having caps on yearly and lifetime payments for health care. Title I of ACA outlaws these business practices. It means that premiums for young adults may be greater than before. The tradeoff is health care that does not lead to increased personal debt. Does ACA policy resolve the barriers ex-perienced by Kathy? Kathy did not attend college and has two dependent children of her own. The proposal for free care for everyone under the age of 30 would have made a difference in Kathy's life. Unfortunately, for her the proposal that would have given free coverage for her sons was not included in the final version of the law.

## SUMMARY

Health behaviors do not completely account for premature disease and death in adulthood. There are periods of loss of health insurance associated with the transitions most adults make—independence, family formation, and entry into the workforce. The stories presented in this chapter show the impact of transition on health care access. ACA contains policies responding to the potential for harm caused by transition. Do these policies completely address the loss of health insurance experienced when moving from dependence to independence? No. In the recession of 2008, an estimated 700,000 to 800,000 persons lost their jobs each month for three consecutive months. Many of these persons had teens in their households who were on the cusp of a young adult transition. There is no national health care policy to provide a bridge for this immediate need. Parents cannot extend coverage if they cannot afford to purchase COBRA. Data from the Bureau of Labor Statistics indicate that only 7 percent of unemployed workers buy into COBRA. An appreciation for the transition experience of young adults requires a complex conversation between two generations to bridge different images of the health care delivery system. Solutions cannot be crafted if the need is not known. The Commonwealth Fund and the Casey Foundation have made a great start toward improving our understanding of transition and health care inequity. Their efforts are not complete unless they spark a conversation between the generation that makes health care policy and the one making the transition. The challenge to effective communication is imagining the unimaginable. Each generation's experience with the system is so different that words cannot begin to capture it. Ask most persons over age 50 to describe the health care system. The version they describe is dated. It contains two parts—a traditional doctor's office and the hospital. When things get out of hand, you rush to the emergency room. Young adults only know the system they see today. For them, reality is a series of around-the-clock choices for outpatient care. These choices include traditional offices, retail clinics, federal clinics, and the local health department. When things get out of hand, you check wait times online for area hospital emergency departments and pick the shortest one. Without a common vision, intergenerational communication is not possible. Without communication, young adults experience health care inequity.

A central theme of this chapter is the idea that health care inequity experienced by young adults progresses to disparity.

Young adults are the nation's most valuable human resource—the workforce, new families, and leadership for the next century. Their tax dollars support public insurance—Medicaid and Medicare. They provide military service in Iraq and Afghanistan. They are stakeholders in the health care delivery system being developed. Yet, their voices were not widely heard during the health reform debate. A fundamental understanding of their experience with insurance loss during the transition to adulthood was absent from our national discussion. At this point, the reader might ask, how is health insurance in young adulthood linked to health disparities? Young adults, after all, have the lowest rates of any disease when compared to other age groups. Young adults have the lowest mortality rates. Young adults rarely come up in discussions of disparities because the language is focused on specific diseases like diabetes and heart attack. These diseases are not common among young adults.

The best measure of health care inequity for young adults is unmet medical need—not disease rates. Difficulty in successfully obtaining health care—however small or large—creates disparity. Health insurance—public or private—is the ticket to health care. In the usual health disparities talk, disadvantage is identified by comparing groups. Sometimes, the speakers forget that no group is immune to disease. Disadvantage means that some just have more disease than others. Excess disease rates for racial groups are readily apparent even at this early stage of life. African American and Hispanic young adults clearly show the signs of disadvantage when compared to white, non-Hispanic, young adults. Economic disadvantage also contributes to differences in disease rates. Among whites, rates are higher for young adults from families with low incomes. If young adult health care access is sensitive to transition, why do we not use *likelihood of transition* as a comparison group? Groups of middle-aged and older adults have fewer transitions. This comparison is one that researchers will need to improve. Better policy will be made when the connection between loss of health insurance, barrier to care, and health disparities is clearly defined.

Transition into the workforce is probably the easiest place to begin looking at the connection between transition and health. Young adults entering the workforce are most sensitive to changes in employer-sponsored health insurance benefits, regulations surrounding preexisting conditions, and the payment process. Currently, the majority of Americans between the ages of 19 and 64 obtain health insurance through the workplace. Individuals who work in small businesses obtain coverage through the individual or small markets. Employment indirectly influences access issues for transitioning young adults. Dependent young adults are typically insured through parental employer-sponsored plans or Medicaid/CHIP. Independent young adults have their own employer-sponsored plans. Employment cycles of boom and bust are disproportionately hardest on both low-seniority workers and transitioning young adults. The Gen X workforce landscape is different from the one encountered by the boomers when they were similarly aged 30 years or more ago. A report prepared by former Labor Secretary, Elaine Chao, describes these differences in the U.S. workforce, its structure, and composition for successive birth cohorts. Gen X and Millennial workers are entering a time where workers are in increasingly short supply. This is one difference from the boomers' experience of a workplace where employers had an excess of workers entering the workforce. This net decline in workforce is leading to changes in the structure of compensation. Employers are planning on being able to count health insurance as part of new compensation schemes for workers in the Gen X and Millennial cohort job market. For boomers, health insurance was tax-free compensation. Gen X and Millennial cohorts will pay taxes on their employer-sponsored plans. They will also be required to choose the package of benefits included in their health plan. Choice can be positive as long as there are a variety of beneficial choices available. Title I of ACA contains an essential benefits clause. This clause creates a minimum standard for health insurance benefits. The mandate of minimum standards prevents the sale of policies with missing health care benefits—like maternity—from being sold. Regulations protecting young adults from the unpleasant surprises of unanticipated injury and unplanned pregnancies are young adult–friendly policies. Essential benefit insurance plans provide minimum health care to meet the needs of transitioning young adults.

The U.S. health care delivery system will continue to offer choices. These choices consist of locations for health care. Convenience is another part of the Gen X and Millennial psychology. Does the ACA change the health care delivery system and improve access through the many portals available? These portals include retail clinics, intermediate care offices, and hospital emergency departments. An emerging business model in the health care delivery system is a clinic with a limited menu of services. These retail clinics are often adjacent to a pharmacy, a grocery store, or a big-box chain store like Wal-Mart. Access to these facilities is simpler than the traditional private practice office. These facilities promote consumer-directed decisions. These facilities are preferred by young adults, families with small children, and middle-aged adults with one or two illnesses or injuries. They are not designed to accommodate persons who are acutely ill with preexisting, multiple medical conditions or functional limitations. Many of these facilities post their prices for minor medical treatments to emphasize low prices and convenience. They do not provide continuity of care that young adults with disabilities may require for independence.

This is an analysis of the ACA and its potential to diminish health care access inequity for young adults. The ACA resolves many of the health care inequities experienced by young adults by creating multiple pathways to both private and public insurance. The idea of multiple paths to insurance may have the greatest impact on disparities created by transitions in young life. Access, not illness, defines disparity among young adults. The high level of vitality and health at this stage of life masks the potential for disparity. History shows us that there is a time lag between inequity and the appearance of disparity. The ACA has the potential to change access inequities that are specific for transitioning young adults—exiting the nest, family formation, and early stage chronic disease. These access inequities have a direct bearing on the current dialogue surrounding Medicaid. Medicaid is the one public plan that comprehensively serves the needs of young adults. Continued support for Medicaid is controversial. Some want to eliminate it altogether. Others want to scale back its services. The ACA has a provision to expand eligibility for childless adults in 2014. Young adults in transition will clearly be disadvantaged by any policy that reduces the size and scope of Medicaid.

There are advocates who envisioned the need for intergenerational consensus in health care. During the Clinton attempt to reform health care, Rosenbaum (1993) called for broad structural support to provide a package of primary care services responsive to the needs of all families—regardless of socioeconomic status. Nancy Henkin (1999) framed this need as intergenerational programming:

we appear to be at a critical juncture in the development of intergenerational programming—one in which careful research and evaluation stand to play a significant role. There is a widespread view . . . that the intergenerational approach to meeting various community needs is on the verge of *going to scale*: becoming integrated into the overall missions of large scale organizations and service delivery systems, especially in the United States. Success in this next level of growth depends on a concerted effort to disseminate what we know about the work we have done. We have learned much over the last twenty years, and providing the best program models for large scale replication depends on documenting our successes and challenges effectively and understanding them fully.

Researchers consistently demonstrate that years of schooling is a key factor influencing health. Years of schooling explains the connection between literacy and health. Education also influences employment prospects. In the United States, 77 percent of workers obtain their health insurance through the workplace. Distinguishing between illiteracy and health care access is important because each requires a very different approach. If education is connected to health through literacy, then public health interventions should focus on reading skills. If, on the other hand, education connects through employer-sponsored health insurance, then interventions should focus on access. We, as a nation, have only one chance to get it right for the current generation of young adults.

## BIBLIOGRAPHY

Asthana, Sheena, and Joyce Halliday. "Developing an Evidence Base for Policies and Interventions to Address Health Inequalities: The Analysis of 'Public Health Regimes.' " *Milbank Quarterly*, no. 3 (2006): 577–603.

Bohmer, Robert. "The Rise of In-Store Clinics—Threat or Opportunity?" *New England Journal of Medicine*, no. 8 (2007): 765–68.

Centers for Disease Control and Prevention. "Trends in Length of Stay for Hospital Deliveries—United States, 1970–1992." *Morbidity and Mortality Weekly Report*, no. 17 (1995): 335–37.

Centers for Medicare & Medicaid Services. "Medicare Program; Clarifying Policies Related to the Responsibilities of Medicare-Participating Hospitals in Treating Individuals with Emergency Medical Conditions." Federal Register CMS-1063-F, 2011.

Collins, Sara R., Jennifer L. Nicholson, and Sheila D. Rustgi. "An Analysis of Leading Congressional Health Care Bills, 2007–2008: Part 1, Insurance Coverage." *Commission on a High Performance System*, no. 1223 (2009): 132pp.

Congressional Research Service. "Americans with Disabilities Act of 1990 as Amended 2008." Public Law 110-325, 2008.

Davis, M. M. "More Children Expected to Seek Care at Retail Clinics." *National Poll on Children's Health*, no. 1 (April 2007): 2pp.

Elo, Irma T., Pekka Martikainen, and Kirsten P. Smith. "Socioeconomic differentials in mortality in Finland and the United States: The Role of Education and Income." *European Journal of Population*, no. 2 (2006): 179–203.

Exworthy, Mark. "Policy to Tackle the Social Determinants of Health: Using Conceptual Models to Understand the Policy Process." *Health Policy and Planning* 23 (2008): 318–27.

Fry-Johnson, Yvonne W., Robert Levine, Diane Rowley, Vincent Agboto, and George Rust. "United States Black: White Infant Mortality Disparities Are Not Inevitable: Identification of Community Resilience Independent of Socioeconomic Status." *Ethnicity & Disease*, no. 20 (Supplement 1) (2010): S131–S35.

Henkin, Nancy. "Forward." *Child and Youth Services* 20, no. 1/2 (1999): xix–xx.

Hogan & Hartson LLP. "President Signs the Pediatric Research Equity Act of 2003 Requiring Specific Assessment of Safety and Efficacy in Children." December 2003, http://www.hoganlovells.com/.

Irvin, Carol, Jeffrey Ballou, and Audra Wenzlow. "Money Follows the Person (MFP): Opportunities for Long-Term Care (LTC) Systems." September 24, 2009, http://www.mathematica-mpr.com/publications.

Jekielek, Susan, and Brett Brown. "The Transition to Adulthood: Characteristics of Young Adults Ages 18 to 24 in America." Census 2000, The Annie E. Casey Foundation, Population Reference Bureau, and Child Trends, May 2005.

Jencks, Christopher. *The Homeless*. Cambridge, MA: Harvard University Press, 1995.

Kaiser Family Foundation and National Women's Law Center. "Women's Access to Care: A State-Level Analysis of Key Health Policies." Vers. 3326. 2003, http://www.kff.org/womenshealth/upload/Full-Report.pdf.

Kaiser Family Foundation and National Women's Law Center. "Medicaid and Children's Health Insurance Program Provisions in the New Health Reform Law." Vers. 7952-03. April 7, 2010, http://www.kff.org/healthreform/upload/7952-03.pdf.

Kentucky Cabinet for Health and Family Services. n.d., http://www.chfs.ky.gov.

Marmot, Michael, Sharon Friel, Ruth Bell, Tanja T. J. Houweling, and Sebastian Taylor. "Closing the Gap in a Generation: Health Equity through Action on the Social Determinants of Health." *The Lancet* 372 (2008): 1661–69.

McDonough, John E., Brian K. Gibbs, Janet L. Scott-Harris, Amanda M. Navarro, Karl Kronebusch, and Kima Taylor. "A State Policy Agenda to Eliminate Racial and Health Disparities." 746, The Commonwealth Fund, 2004.

McWilliams, Michael J. "Health Consequences of Uninsurance among Adults in the United States: Recent Evidence and Implications." *The Millbank Quarterly* 87, no. 2 (2009): 443–94.

Mehrotra, A., M. C. Wang, J. Adams, J. R. Lave, and E. A. McGlynn. "Retail Clinics, Primary Care Physicians, and Emergency Departments: A Comparison of Patient Visits." *Health Affairs* 27, no. 5 (2008): 1272–82.

Murray, Christopher J. L., Sandeep C. Kulkarni, Catherine Michaud, Niels Tomihima Niels, Maria T. Bulzacchelli, Terrell J. Landiorio, and Majid Ezzati. "Eight Americas: Investigating Mortality Disparities across Races,

Counties, and Race-Counties in the United States." *PLoS Medicine*. September 12, 2006, http://www.plosmedicine.org/article/info:doi/10.1371/journal.pmed.0030260.

National Alliance on Mental Illness and Public Policy Institute. "Impact and Cost of Mental Illness: The Case of Bipolar Disorder." National Alliance on Mental Illness. n.d., http://www.nami.org/Content/NavigationMenu/Inform_Yourself/About_Public_Policy/Policy_Research_Institute/Policymakers_Toolkit/Impact_and_Cost_of_Mental_Illness_Bipolar.htm.

National Institutes of Health. "Best Pharmaceuticals for Children Act (BPCA) Priority List of Needs in Pediatric Therapeutics." *Federal Register* 68, no. 13 (2003): 2789–90. Revised version *Federal Register* 74, no. 70 (2009): 17203–05.

Nicholson, Jennifer L., and Sara R. Collins. "Young, Uninsured, and Seeking Change: Health Coverage of Young Adults and Their Views on Health Reform." Vers. 73. The Commonwealth Fund, December 2009, http://www.commonwealthfund.org/Newsletters/The-Commonwealth-Fund-Connection/2009/December-18-2009/Whats-New/Young-Uninsured-and-Seeking-Change-Health-Coverage-of-Young-Adults-and-Their-Views-on-Health-Reform.aspx.

Nicholson, Jennifer L., Sara R. Collins, Sara R. Mahato, Elise Bisundev-Gould, Cathy Schoen, and Shelia D. Rustgi. "Right of Passage? Why Young Adults Become Uninsured and How New Policies Can Help, 2009 Update." Vers. 22. The Commonwealth Fund, 2009, http://www.commonwealthfund.org/Publications/Issue-Briefs/2009/Aug/Rite-of-Passage-Why-Young-Adults-Become-Uninsured-and-How-New-Policies-Can-Help-2009-Update.aspx.

Niederdeppe, Jeff Q., Lisa Blu, Porismita Borah, David A. Kindig, and Stephanie A. Robert. "Message Design Strategies to Raise Public Awareness of Social Determinants of Health and Population Health Disparities." *The Millbank Quarterly* 86, no. 3 (2008): 481–513.

O'Hare, William P. *Kids Count Data Book*. ISSN 1060-9814, The Annie E. Casey Foundation, 2004.

Patient Protection and Affordable Care Act of 2010. Public Law 111-148, U.S. Statutes at Large, 2010, 124 Stat. 119.

Paulin, Geoffrey D. "Examining Expenditure Patterns of Young Single Adults in a Historical Context." *Consumer Expenditure Survey Anthology*, 52–73, 2008.

Paulin, Geoffrey D. "Expenditure Patterns of Young Single Adults: Two Recent Generations Compared." *Monthly Labor Review* 131, no. 12 (2008): 19–51.

Paulin, Geoffrey D., and Brian Riodon. "Making It on Their Own: The Baby Boom Meets Generation X." *Monthly Labor Review* 131, no. 13 (1998): 10–21.

Paulin, Geoffrey D., and Elizabeth M. Dietz. "Health Insurance Coverage for Families with Children: Findings from the Consumer Expenditure Survey." Abbreviated from Monthly Labor Review. U.S. Bureau of Labor. 1995, http://www.bls.gov/ore/pdf/st950150.pdf.

Picket, Kate. "Questions and Answer: Howard Dean on the Politics of Health Care Reform." *Time* magazine. Published electronically July 21, 2009, http://www.time.com/time/nation/article/0,8599,1911849,00.html.

Ranji, Usha, Aline Salganicoff, Alexandra M. Stewart, Marisa Cox, and Lauren Doamekpor. "State Medicaid Coverage of Perinatal Services: Summary of State Survey Findings." Publication no. 8014, Kaiser Family Foundation and The George Washington University School of Public Health and Health Services, 2009.

Rosenbaum, Sara. "Providing Primary Health Care to Children: Integrating Primary Care Services with Health Insurance Principles." *The Future of Children* 3, no. 2 (1993): 60–76.

Rossi, Peter H. *Down and Out in America: The Origins of Homelessness*. Chicago: University of Chicago Press, 1989.

Rudavsky, R., and R. Mehrotra. "Sociodemographic Characteristics of Communities Served by Retail Clinics." *Journal of the American Board of Family Medicine* 23, no. 1 (2010): 42–48.

Schrammel, Kurt. "Comparing the Labor Market Success of Young Adults from Two Generations." *Monthly Labor Review* 23, no. 1 (1998): 3–9.

Scott, M. K. *Health Care in the Express Lane: The Emergence of Retail Clinics*. Oakland, CA: California HealthCare Foundation, 2006.

Scott, M. K. *Health Care in the Express Lane: Retail Clinics Go Mainstream*. Oakland, CA: California HealthCare Foundation, 2007.

Shih, Anthony, Karen Davis, Stephen C. Schoenbaum, Anne Gauthier, Rachel Nuzum, and Douglas McCarthy. "Organizing the United States Health Care Delivery System for High Performance." Publication no. 1155, The Commonwealth Fund, 2008.

Smedley, Brian D. "Moving beyond Access: Achieving Equity in State Health Care Reform." *Health Affairs* 27, no. 2 (2008): 447–55.

Starfield, Barbara, Leiyu Sheu, and James Macinko. "Contribution of Primary Care to Health Systems and Health." *Milbank Quarterly* 83, no. 3 (2005): 457–502.

Sum, Andrew, and Ishwar Khatiwada. "The Nation's Underemployed in the 'Great Recession' of 2007–09." *Monthly Labor Review* 133, no. 11 (2010): 3–15.

Texas Children's Health Plan. n.d., http://www.texaschildrenshealthplan.org.

Udom, Nduka U., and Charles L. Betley. "Effects of Maternity-Stay Legislation on Drive-through Deliveries." *Health Affairs* 17, no. 3 (1998): 208–15.

U.S. Congress, 107th. "Americans with Disabilities Act of 1990 as Amended 2008." United States Statutes at Large, 2002, 115 Stat. 1408.

U.S. Congress, 108th. "H.R.1 Medicare Prescription Drug, Improvement and Modernization Act of 2003." DOCID: f:publ173.108, 2003, Public Law 108-173.

U.S. Department of Labor. Bureau of Labor Statistics. "On Benefits by Wage Level: Survey Finds that Employer-Provided Benefits Vary with Earnings."

*Program Perspectives* 2, no. 1 (2010), http://www.bls.gov/opub/perspectives/program_perspectives_vol2_issue1.pdf.

U.S. Department of Labor. "Persons with a disability: Labor Force Characteristics." USDL-11-0921, June 2011.

U.S. Department of Labor. "Usual Weekly Earnings of Wage and Salary Workers—2nd Quarter 2011." No. USDL-11-10-1082, July 2011.

U.S. Department of Labor. Employee Benefit Security Administration (EBSA). "An Employee's Guide to Health Benefits under COBRA: The Consolidated Omnibus Budget Reconciliation Act." n.d., http://www.dol.gov/ebsa.

U.S. Equal Employment Opportunity Commission. "Facts About Pregnancy Discrimination." n.d., http://www.eeoc.gov/facts/fs-preg.html.

U.S. Government Accountability Office. "Stronger Department of Education Oversight Needed to Help Ensure Only Eligible Students Receive Federal Student Aid." Report to the Chairman, Subcommittee on Higher Education, Lifelong Learning, & Competitiveness, Committee on Education & Labor, House of Representatives. GAO-09-600, 2009.

U.S. Internal Revenue Service. "Health Savings Accounts and Other Tax-Favored Health Plans." November 25, 2009, http://www.irs.gov/pub/irs-pdf/p969.pdf.

Walker, James A. "Employment Characteristics of Gulf War-Era II Veterans in 2006: A Visual Essay." *Monthly Labor Review*, no. 11 (May 2008): 3–13.

Wright, James D. *Address Unknown: The Homeless in America*. Hawthorne, NY: Aldine de Gruyter, 1989.

Yi, Song G. "Consumer-Driven Health Care: What Is It and What Does It Mean for Employees and Employers?" Compensation and Working Conditions online, U.S. Department of Labor, Bureau of Labor Statistics, October 25, 2010.

# CHAPTER 8

## Correctable Disparity, the Affordable Care Act, and Public Health Research

Our ability to identify and change the landscape of health disparity is a direct result of scientific research. One by-product of the Affordable Care Act will be public health research that will help address the problem of health disparities. Researchers pursue several different lines of inquiry. Biomedical researchers tend to focus on individual characteristics. These include behavior, biological traits, and in some studies exposure to environmental toxins. These researchers tend to ignore the contribution of legislation on their conclusions about the source of population differences in diseases. Social scientists can frame disparities as a resource issue. Missing access to societal capital—education, opportunities, and financial resources are common points of study. There are also studies of social welfare. Programs with early childhood supports like Head Start have been evaluated for their impact on future success in school. Somewhere in the published reports from these studies, a statement alludes to barriers in health care access. Some researchers define this barrier as an individual decision that delays care seeking. Others define the barrier as missing financial resources to pay for health care. There is little commentary raising the possibility of well-intentioned but poor quality care or the possibility of fraudulent services.

Health care is an interaction between the individual and the delivery system. If we are serious about eliminating health disparities, then we also need research that incorporates the appearance of new laws. Research redesign is not easy. Scientists are well known for extended debate about best practices. Right now, many do not see a direct connection between their own research and the data available from ACA. What does the Consumer Assessment of Healthcare Providers and Systems survey have to do with a clinical trial of some new surgical procedure? Does the compliance of a local health care delivery system with the Cultural and Linguistically Appropriate Standards influence recruitment of participants in a community-based research project? How can we connect headlines reporting a billion dollar settlement for health care fraud to the prior five years of death and illness in the area where it happened? These are the questions that can be answered by health disparity researchers.

To incorporate this new approach to the existing research, we need the idea of *correctable disparities*. Correctable disparities are measurable differences that decline with system changes. The Center for Studying Health System Change (CSHSC) has been a thought leader in this area. *Avoidable hospitalizations, patient activation,* and *ambulatory care–sensitive conditions* are measurements routinely used in CSHSC analyses. Each one incorporates the idea of an interaction between patient and health care delivery system. In this final chapter, I will look back at some of my own publications. What does the passage of ACA do to alter the central question, the core design, or the interpretation of the results? If disparities are to be resolved, then researchers must develop the language of correctable disparities.

## DISPARITY: CANCER AND OLDER MINORITIES

The work of a gerontologist places us in a position to see the impact of health care inequity on health and vitality in late life. Public health research in gerontology has a central focus on living longer. It is not enough, however, to achieve old age. The holy grail of aging research is staying well and preserving functional capacity. In 2005, I published an analysis of the challenge that cancer presents for older adults. At that time, the report examined three areas of cancer care that could be addressed with policy changes. The cancer care policies in place at the time limited early detection, treatment, and rehabilitation during the cancer recovery phase for older adults. To identify correctable disparities in racial and ethnicity cancer death, I proposed that our understanding of cancer disparities could be improved with an evaluation of regional variation in cancer screening among Medicare beneficiaries. The Aligning Forces for Quality group—collaboration between the Robert Wood Johnson Foundation and the Dartmouth group—also saw the need for analyses of regional variation. Their reports focused on preventive services for diabetes care among Medicare beneficiaries. They found evidence of missing preventive care, rates of hospitalization, and high cost of health care. To illustrate the issues surrounding minority elders and ACA, let us consider the sources of health care inequities surrounding cancer screening and care.

Primary care practices have a role in cancer diagnosis and care disparities. Physician recommendation is the most important factor in cancer screening. This means that screening may not take place despite access to care. Physicians report that they often do not discuss cancer screening tests with their patients. Other factors, like limited examination time and language barriers, are associated with a low probability of discussion about cancer screening. Physician belief in the value of specific tests and his or her intention to order tests can be associated with probability of discussion about the pros and cons of cancer screening. Physician bias may cause some patients to be inappropriately denied the opportunity to choose whether to screen for prostate cancer. Clinical guidelines make a vague reference to life expectancy of less than 10 years but do not offer more explicit guidance to either physician or patient. All of these factors have the potential significantly to influence the experience of minority elders with cancer screening. The new data collection guidelines in ACA give researchers a line of sight into smaller units of health care delivery. Is there bias in practice? Is this preference for treatment based on evidence? Can we detect provider bias accompanied by excess mortality and morbidity?

What about older minorities who are cancer survivors and the primary care practices caring for these survivors? Does their history of cancer create access barriers? Counting the number of cancer survivors is one way to see the aftercare experience of minorities. Prevalence is statistic used by researchers to account for the number of survivors. With this measure, primary care providers can see the total volume of cancer survivors in the pool of patients served by their practice. Many primary care practices were blind to the total number of cancer survivors in their practices. ACA and the American Revitalization and Reinvestment Act, also known as the Stimulus (Public Law 111-09), reward primary care practices that make meaningful use of electronic health records. Health care planning and resource allocation represent an important practical application of prevalence estimates. Most importantly, prevalence data can be used to identify concerns unique to cancer survivors within the panel. Correcting disparities begins with the infrastructure to measure the variety of medical conditions served within an individual primary care practice.

To dig a little further into the data issue, let us examine the statistical measures needed to accurately estimate cancer prevalence for minorities.

How do researchers make this measurement? Does ACA improve the detail in the data? Prevalence is defined as the number or percentage of people in a population alive on a certain date who were previously diagnosed with the disease. Prevalence includes new (incidence) plus additional preexisting cases. It is determined largely by past incidence and survival. Most cross-sectional studies, such as the National Health Interview Survey, the National Health Examination and Nutritional Survey, the Behavioral Risk Factor Surveillance Survey, and the National Ambulatory Medical Care Survey, report prevalence data for a variety of chronic diseases along with medical outcomes, such as history of cancer. These surveys form the bedrock of our understanding of health disparities. These are samples of patients. The surveys tell us very little about the health care delivery systems in which minorities receive their care. As cancer survival has improved, both public health advocates and cancer survivors have expressed interest in measuring cancer prevalence. Statistical problems of estimating cancer prevalence are an area of active inquiry. The Connecticut Tumor Registry, Surveillance Epidemiology and End Results Program, and EUROPRE-VAL provide the underlying data for most of these studies. The Surveillance Epidemiology and End Results Program have gone the extra step of collecting data for minority populations in select areas of the United States. None of the U.S. registries provides complete coverage of the population. Reported prevalence rates from each of these studies cannot be directly compared because different standard populations are used to age-adjust the samples. Each estimate is based on a 1 to 5 percent sample of adults. Prevalence estimates from registry data are limited. Sometimes the individual registry patient cannot be found. This is particularly true with minorities. In the 1970s when the National Cancer Institute began its work toward measuring cancer among U.S. minorities, these were the kinds of issues under consideration. ACA policy builds on this experience.

Before the Surveillance Epidemiology and End Results Program, prevalence of cancer was estimated using single-time surveys. The surveys tell you who has survived cancer. Byrne and colleagues used the National Health Interview Survey, Cancer Control Supplement, or the Epidemiology Supplement to estimate cancer prevalence. In this survey, the participant was asked "Has a physician ever told you that you have cancer?" They reported that the most common cancer sites (prostate, breast, and colon) were comparable with the Surveillance Epidemiology and End Results Program incidence series. Second, they reported that *prevalence rates* were higher for whites than for blacks. This racial prevalence difference is the flip side of the relative disparity in survival of whites compared to blacks. Third, the surveys clearly show that cancer prevalence rates increase with older age. For example, almost 40 percent of people aged 75 and older had a history of a cancer diagnosis. Fourth, among those who said they had a first cancer, 8 percent reported having had a second cancer. A similar estimate for occurrence of a second tumor from Surveillance Epidemiology and End Results Program data suggests that approximately 20 percent of older adult cancer survivors have developed a new primary cancer site. The National Health Interview Survey excludes people living in institutions, so it is not known whether older cancer patients or cancer survivors are overrepresented in nursing homes. The National Health Interview Survey is a national probability survey designed to generate population-based prevalence rates for the United States, whereas Surveillance Epidemiology and End Results Program is a geographically limited cancer registry. Persons who reported a history of cancer in National Health Interview Survey cannot be verified with histologic confirmation of a case. Verifying an individual's history of cancer using tumor registry data is a labor-intensive process. It requires a high fidelity of information between tumor registries and persons reporting a history of cancer. These findings suggest, however, that primary care practices with disproportionate numbers of elderly whites are most likely to have the highest cancer prevalence rates. Reports of cancer history—prevalent cancer cases in primary care practices—can be verified in Surveillance Epidemiology and End Results Program data only if the practice is located in the same geographic region as the registry.

The experience of cancer survivors might be best understood within the context of primary care practices. Within practices, there is considerable clustering by race, ethnicity, income, and age. For example, practices within urban areas have greater proportions of African Americans in their panels simply because the overall geographic density is greater. U.S. physicians who work in these settings conduct their medical practices knowing that black men in the United States have a higher incidence of prostate cancer and higher mortality rate from the disease. Low income and advanced age are two other risk factors for prostate cancer. There is clustering within practices of these traits. There are financially disadvantaged primary practices serving African Americans. These practices lack adequate access to diagnostic technologies used in cancer screening for colorectal, prostate, and breast cancer. These practice-level differences in access to diagnostic technology and its relationship to population distribution are potentially a major contributing factor in higher advanced-stage cancer incidence, lower prevalence, and diminished survival. There is also evidence indicating clustering within primary care practices of cancer survivors. Since the development of these surveys, legislation has changed the eligibility of older adults for clinical trials and payment for physician-initiated goals-of-care conversations. What can the new data available in ACA tell us about these critical parts of the care for older adult cancer survivors?

As discussed in the previous chapters, the mortality experience in the United States can be subdivided into "Eight Americas." These groups include racial and ethnic minorities, persons with less than a high school education, persons clustered in specific geographic regions, and members of households that are supported by low-wage jobs. Barriers in access to health care make a substantial contribution to this excess death and disability. Ever-increasing numbers of the U.S. middle class are experiencing this specific barrier. Indeed, this collective experience was the political force driving the legislative efforts culminating in the ACA. A central theme of this chapter is that health disparity researchers need to shift the frame from *individual experience* of disease to a frame that includes both the *individual* and the *system of health care*. When the *individual* occupies the entire frame, the main product of health disparity studies can be classified in three ways. There are studies that document the size of the gap between groups. These studies serve a witness function. At the end of the study, there is usually a statement like "Blacks experience greater rates than other groups and more research is needed to identify causal factors." Other studies seek to define causal factors and can be thought of as etiology studies. The summary statement for this research can be paraphrased as follows "Individual genetic effects may account for higher rates of diabetes." A third variety of studies focuses on a specific factor and the attempt to measure its effectiveness on an individual. These studies typically end with a statement like "Our approach improves individual adherence to the treatment among Hispanics." A frame that includes both the *individual* and the *delivery system* of health care could serve all the functions described—witness, etiology, and treatment effectiveness assessment. The design, however, could estimate the impact of systemic factors.

## DISPARITY CANCER, OLDER MINORITIES, AND ACA-MODIFIED RECOMMENDATIONS

In 2005, I proposed a series of recommendations to decrease cancer disparities among minority elders. The recommendations were not designed to be comprehensive. Rather, they were proposed to evoke further thinking by the larger community of public health researchers. ACA has made new tools available for researchers to extend the process of designing correctable disparity research. The climate surrounding cancer treatment for older adults and payment for their participation in clinical trials has also evolved. In the current climate for prostate cancer detection and treatment, racial and ethnic disparities continue to exist. However, Medicare payment policy has changed. Let us revisit the recommendations to see whether new opportunities have emerged. One new opportunity rests with the availability of electronic health records. Researchers have suspected that there is regional variation in the cancer risk associated with a PSA value. Does a level of five mg/dl carry the same probability of significant prostate cancer in San Antonio, Texas, as it does in Washington, DC? With electronic record linkage, health care systems can aggregate *all* PSA test results. Risk for underlying prostate cancer can be evaluated within the context community norms. By assigning risk within a regional context, small area variation in population disease can be appreciated. This use of small area variation to enhance interpretation of PSA test results will improve application of care until a more sensitive test comes along. Small area variation can be detected with the ACA emphasis on data collection. This approach to quality improvement was used by the Veterans Health Administration. Understanding variation in a small area created a climate that led to its current placement at the top of the U.S. health care system.

Some correctable causes of health disparities required a specific focus on outpatient primary care practice. One recommendation included *ensuring that all primary care practices have access to cancer diagnostic and treatment facilities*. ACA does not have specific language linking each primary care practice to cancer diagnostic and treatment facilities. Correcting this source of health care access inequity will need continued monitoring. Another primary care practice issue relates to the factors influencing differences in physician cancer screening patterns. The combined ACA emphasis on quality and the delivery of preventive services will create opportunities for researchers to define sources of bias in practice patterns related to race, age, and functional status of patients. Identifying and supporting primary care practices with disproportionate numbers of cancer survivors will be possible with the advent of ACA payment policies that encourage the use of electronic health records. These practices are also most likely to provide care to persons with fewer economic and social resources. Are the practices themselves disadvantaged by the lack of income and forced to provide fewer services? What can health policy do to assist these practices as they meet the needs of an increasingly older adult population?

## REGIONAL VARIATION IN PREVENTIVE CARE AND OLDER MINORITIES: EXPANDED REFERENCE FRAME

To illustrate a starting place for this expanded frame of reference, consider the problem of health disparities in the Medicare population. The Medicare database clearly shows evidence of regional variation in medical practice. How much of this variation contributes to health disparities? This question extends the frame of reference for health care inequity research. With this perspective, researchers could measure correctable disparities. How much of the size of the gap between the group with the best outcomes and the one with the worst outcomes is caused by the structure of a health care delivery system? In chapter 6, we discussed data from the Dartmouth group demonstrating that blacks and whites in Mississippi with diabetes had similar rates of lower limb amputation. Moreover, whites in Mississippi were more likely to have a lower limb amputation than whites in Utah. This example illustrates the complexity of health disparities in the United States. Race and region of residence clearly interact to influence the probability of losing a limb.

Current policy research is focused exclusively on Medicare spending and system financing. Is there evidence of health care inequalities in a population with access to health care? Can the Medicare population provide a starting place to examine the connection between health disparities and the reformation of health care to improve access, lower cost, and improve quality? Medicare is a federal health insurance program for 45 million elderly and disabled Americans. What role does Medicare play in either creating or attenuating health disparities? Medicare helps to pay for hospital and physician visits, prescription drugs, and other health care services. Dual eligible beneficiaries—persons simultaneously enrolled in Medicare and Medicaid—form a cohort of the nation's most vulnerable older adults. This population is defined by its low income. More than 61 percent live on an annual income of less than 10,000 dollars. Although some members of this cohort have engaged in a spend-down process to become eligible for Medicaid-supported long-term care, it is likely that most dual eligible beneficiaries have lived with lifelong socioeconomic disadvantage. What would the health disparity research frame look like for older adults who are dual eligible? With the new data requirements of ACA, researchers will be able to monitor quality of care for the dual eligibles and disabled persons supported by Medicaid.

Enter Medicare into a search engine and more than 90 percent of the research reports retrieved will focus on one of two areas: costs of services or system financing. The frames of reference are factors that drive health care consumption and pricing. Reports that are concerned with financing focus on the stability of the Medicare Trust Fund. There is no mention of health disparities or economically disadvantaged elders. The Bureau of Economic Analyses created a website to showcase its research to develop new indices for pricing health care (see http://www.bea.gov/national/health_care_satellite_account.htm). Cost control, not population level access, is the main focus of this site. A discussion of health disparities does not appear in reports that evaluate the profitability of a hospital or other health care provider. See the report that U.S. hospitals experienced zero profit margins during the first quarter of 2009. Few studies have examined health disparities with a specific focus on Medicare beneficiaries. Skinner and Zhou (2006) have proposed several strategies for measuring trends in health disparity in this specific group. Among the measures they propose are expenditures and their link to age-specific life expectancy. Their analyses provide compelling evidence that when Medicare beneficiaries are stratified by income, there are striking disparities in *expenditures*. These differentials in expenditures are significantly correlated with gaps in life expectancy. In other words, low-income Medicare beneficiaries have lower per capita expenditures and lower life expectancies.

Regional variation in both disease and Medicare expenditures is another potential starting point for health disparity research. The Dartmouth Atlas Project (DAP) is a claims database. It comes from the Centers for Medicare and Medicaid Services (CMS). This federal agency collects data for every person and provider using Medicare health insurance. Access to these data is made available for research purposes. See http://www.dartmouthatlas.org/tools/faq for a full discussion of the sampling frame and other details. Other data sources used to develop this resource include Bureau of the U.S. Census, the American Hospital Association, American Medical Association, National Center for Health Statistics, and Claritas, Incorporated. What does the Dartmouth data tell us about health disparities? Reports using these data show regional variation in Medicare payments (http://www.dartmouthatlas.org/data/region).

There is a paradoxical relationship between Medicare expenditures and quality care measures. In general, regions with the highest Medicare expenditures have the lowest use of preventive services. The Dartmouth Atlas of

Health Care has analyzed Medicare claims data to illustrate this paradox. They show data derived from 306 hospital referral regions. Hospital referral regions are a grouping that contains at least one hospital that performs major cardiac procedures and neurosurgery. For more details describing the definition of hospital referral regions, see http://www.dartmouthatlas. org/data/region. Each area was ranked based on a standardized per capita Medicare expenditure. From 1 to 10, the regions with the highest rates of expenditures include Miami, Florida; McAllen, Texas; Bronx, New York; Manhattan, New York; Harlingen, Texas; Los Angeles, California; East Long Island, New York; Dearborn, Michigan; and Chicago, Illinois. The final rank is further determined by the expenditures *after* the data were adjusted for population differences in age, gender composition, and racial and ethnic differences. This adjustment removes biases associated with advanced age, gender differences in patterns of illness, and severity of illness within racial and ethnic groups. The list does not change much. Miami, Florida, and McAllen, Texas, retain the top two slots. The next eight include Harlingen, Texas; Monroe, Louisiana; Alexandria, Louisiana; Elyria, Ohio; Corpus Christi, Texas; Shreveport, Louisiana; Slidell, Louisiana; and Fort Lauderdale, Florida. These areas have the highest rates of hospital discharge for ambulatory care–sensitive conditions. Ambulatory care–sensitive condition is a correctable indicator of health care inequity. High rates of hospitalization for these illnesses are interpreted as a failure of adequate disease control. This category includes chronic medical conditions such as asthma, diabetes, and congestive heart failure. Low rates of preventive care in these regions can be seen in the percent of diabetics receiving regular eye examinations and the percent with evidence of well-controlled blood sugar (hemoglobin A1C). Most of these areas are well below the national percent for eye examinations (68%) and controlled blood sugar (80%).

The paradox is reinforced with the hospital discharge data for ambulatory care–sensitive conditions in the bottom 10 hospital referral regions. Regions with the lowest hospital discharge rates have the highest use of diabetes-preventive services. These regions include Anchorage, Alaska; Rapid City, South Dakota; Medford, Oregon; Yakima, Washington; Lebanon, New Hampshire; Grand Junction, Colorado; Eugene, Oregon; Salem, Oregon; La Crosse, Wisconsin; and Honolulu, Hawaii. These areas have the lowest rates of hospital discharge for ambulatory care–sensitive conditions. High rates of preventive care in these regions can be seen in the percent of diabetics receiving regular eye examinations and the percent with evidence of well-controlled blood sugar (hemoglobin A1C). In most of these areas, 80 percent or more of their Medicare beneficiaries with diabetes have well-controlled blood sugars.

One unanswered question in health disparity research involves the influence of Medicare policies on health disparities and the impact of disparities on regional variation in costs. Some areas have persistent disparities in health, more disease, and higher death rates. Medicare policies recognize the added costs associated with health disparities. A portion of enrollee Medicare expenditures reflect the costs of caring for a higher number of patients who are older and sicker by recognizing the payments related to *diagnostic-related group*. Another portion of the cost is determined by policies recognizing that many hospitals provide uncompensated care. *Medicare disproportionate share hospitals* care for large numbers of minority elders and also serve large numbers of persons without health insurance. Since 1981, federal law requires state Medicaid programs to take into account the circumstances of hospitals serving a disproportionate number of low-income patients when setting payment rates for inpatient hospital services. Over the past two decades, this requirement has led to the emergence of the Medicaid disproportionate share hospital programs in many states. As was discussed in chapter 2, Medicare disproportionate share hospital payment will change with ACA. This causes concern among health disparity researchers.

Medicare is a major supporter of education. Some areas of the United States have more medical schools than others. Medical schools, however, are not the equivalent of graduate physician training programs. Graduate training refers to the training a physician receives after graduating from medical school. This process takes three to seven years. During training, a resident physician is paid a salary ranging from 40,000 to 60,000 dollars. *Graduate medical education* salaries are paid on a formula that includes salary for the individual physician trainee plus costs to accommodate the inefficiencies associated with training in a clinical setting. Inefficiencies include longer hospital stays, increased medical testing, and lower patient volume per physician. There is regional variation in the distribution of graduate medical education funds because almost 50 percent of all medical residency training slots are located in the northeastern region. The number of residency slots funded by Medicare has been limited to approximately 19,000 since 1997. There are shortages of physicians in many of the areas where the highest spending regions are located. Perhaps, more physicians in these areas would increase competition and lower health care costs.

Does Medicare policy contribute to health disparities? We could also ask the question: "Do any of the additional dollars contribute to higher quality of care?" Patients in the lowest-cost areas are less likely to be hospitalized for a chronic condition. Persons with diabetes in these areas are more likely to get preventative care. Regular eye examinations prevent blindness. Regular HA1c checks to determine long-term control of blood sugar. Control of blood sugar is a sure strategy to prevent the complications of diabetes—heart attack, stroke, blindness, amputation, and premature disability. The Dartmouth Atlas data tells us that policies promoting quality care will lower costs for all regions. The Atlas, however, does not account for factors that contribute to underlying poor health in the population.

Health disparities are both social and political issues as well as public health concerns. Health care reform legislation creates a unique opportunity for social scientists to explicitly access changes in the statistical measures of health disparities. The challenge is linking legislative efforts to correct the system with changes in metrics of health. How can we identify beneficial effects of newly enacted reform measures as well as identify the unintended consequences policy? What kinds of study designs will generate answers that have a direct application to political and public health officials as well as driving social science research? The health care reform efforts present both an opportunity to improve and a risk of exacerbating existing health disparities in the United States. Are there cases from our history that can help rapidly identify unintended consequences? Can prior legislative efforts specifically designed to improve health care provide guidance to researchers and public health officials? By extending the analyses of Medicare expenditures beyond the usual focus on cost containment, health disparity researchers can develop a nuanced view of the causes of and cures for health disparities in late life.

## HEALTH DISPARITY, LEGISLATION, AND PUBLIC HEALTH RESEARCH

The primary product of the legislative process is a new law. How would a public health researcher connect a newly enacted law to indices of death and illness? Analyses of laws and their impact on society are classically the province of legal scholars and historians. The tools employed by these researchers are not familiar to most of the public health research community. For example, legal scholars rely on court cases and develop their analyses from a case-by-case review of court rulings. Historians are probably the most fortunate of all scholars. They have the gift of being able to operate with hindsight. Timelines of 50 to 100 years are ideal for historical analyses. Neither legal scholars nor historians routinely utilize the types of statistical tools that public health uses to measure health disparities. Laws and historical documents do not provide the level of accounting required for quantitative analyses of health disparities used in public health research. How does the current health care reform create opportunities for more direct measures—allowing public health researchers to directly measure the connection between newly enacted legislation and population level trends in morbidity and mortality? Bio-historical analysis is one approach used to link historical events with public health problems occurring over time and geographic distance. This technique of linking historical public health datasets with demographic and historical events is relatively new. Its application to health disparity research is still under development. The remainder of this chapter presents specific research questions that can be used to design studies and facilitate this linkage. This segment is designed to illustrate a new integrated approach for health disparity research.

## Public Law 79-725: The Hill Burton Hospital Survey and Construction Act of 1946

Throughout the text, this law was referenced. In the post–World War II era, it represents a significant beginning of a history of federal direction in the health care infrastructure of the United States. This law was not enacted, as it is sometimes proposed, to desegregate U.S. hospitals during the era of Jim Crow medicine. The Hill Burton Act was designed to provide federal assistance for the planning, construction, and improvement of health care facilities. Recipients of these funds were obligated to provide a minimum dollar amount of *uncompensated care* to individuals who could not pay for medical care. This minimum dollar was based on a formula included in the legislation that accounted for operating costs. The length of time that the facility was obligated to provide free care was based on the type of monies the jurisdiction received. Those facilities receiving loans were obligated until the loan was repaid. Facilities receiving grants were obligated into perpetuity. This act provided support to build or renovate many of the public hospitals across the United States. In 2009, there were 217 Hill Burton obligated facilities nationwide. There are no obligated facilities in Indiana, Nebraska, Nevada, Rhode Island, Utah, and Wyoming. In many areas of the country, the Hill Burton obligated facilities are outpatient clinics or nursing homes. Very few of the remaining services include hospitals. This lack of full-service health care presents a significant barrier for rural communities as well as under-resourced urban areas. A complete list of these facilities can be found on the Health and Human Services website (http://www.hrsa.gov/gethealthcare/affordable/hillburton). For a detailed discussion of the place Hill Burton obligated facilities occupy in the biomedical history of the United States, see Byrd and Clayton (2002). Wailoo (2001) also provides a lively presentation of the process surrounding implementation of Hill Burton legislation in Memphis, Tennessee, during the 1940s and 1950s.

Legislation is not made in a vacuum. It evolves out of a combination of perceived need, envisioned solution, and political will. Just enacting federal law is no guarantee that a need will be addressed. Once legislation is made into law, it can still be stymied by challenges through the court system. The new law takes on a life of its own. In our democracy, a law's effectiveness is still dependent on a consensus process. If passage is marked by a contentious process, then the process of law-initiated change will require continued expenditures of energy by its supporters. If the passage is the result of a broad consensus, then the process of change will begin with broad base of local support. Local concerns, however, will still require attention from proponents of the new law. These concerns carry the potential to distort the original intent of the law. This distortion has the potential to diminish effective application to the need it was designed to resolve in the first place. Hill Burton represented a convergence of opinion that the federal government had a role in making health care available to a broad group of citizens. There was also consensus that the federal government could play a role in this process by making grants and loans available to local communities for the construction of facilities.

The Hill Burton Act is useful to illustrate the differences between health disparity researchers and their frame of reference. Those who use *individual experience* to frame their research might view the history surrounding Hill Burton in the following way: "Hill Burton, enacted in 1946, is an historical event. It is irrelevant to the measurement of mortality and morbidity rates in 2011." Disparity researchers, who combine the individual and the system in a research frame, will understand that new questions and designs immediately come into view. The researchable unit becomes the *individual and Hill Burton obligated facilities.* Across the United States there are 217 facilities that are currently designated as Hill Burton obligated. Does their geographic placement contribute significantly to the variation observed in health disparity statistics across areas? This is particularly important for older adults, Medicaid, and long-term care facilities. Since the 1960s, the number of Hill Burton obligated facilities has declined. Using time trend modeling methods, can we detect an association between these declining numbers and changes in infant mortality and maternal mortality? Simple counts are one approach to measuring Hill Burton facilities. Per capita expenditures in each Hill Burton facility is another approach to measuring the resources available to these facilities. Historical appropriations data for Hill Burton facilities is available through congressional records. Over time, does declining appropriations account for significant variation within a community in mortality and morbidity for users of the Hill Burton facilities? These simple questions create points of collaboration between legislative initiatives and public health models of health disparity research.

## Public Law 100-713: Indian Health Care Amendments (1988)

The role of the U.S. federal government in Indian Health Services is an issue dating back to 1789, when the Department of War was put in charge by Congress to handle Indian Affairs. No one in health disparity research understands this history. Roger Walke has written extensive reports on this history for the Congressional Research Service. Much of this analysis is based on his writings. In 1789, care was provided in the Indian Health Service by military doctors. The earliest Indian treaty providing for health services was signed in 1832 with the Winnebago of Wisconsin (7 Stat. 370). Overall, Congress made 44 treaty commitments to provide tribes with a physician, a hospital, medicines, or vaccine, or some combination of these resources. Many of the treaties contained a delimited time. The Snyder Act of 1921 provides basic authorization for Indian health care without time or dollar limitations. It authorized the Bureau of Indian Affairs to "direct, supervise, and expend such moneys as Congress may from time to time appropriate, for the benefit, care, and assistance of the Indians . . . for relief of distress." The Indian Health Care Improvement Act of 1976, as amended through 2000, Public Law 94-437, was enacted to provide "the highest possible health status to Indians and to provide existing Indian Health Services with all the resources necessary to effect that policy." Some of the specific goals of the act were "to increase the number of Indian health professionals, to eliminate deficiencies in health status and resources, to improve health facilities, and to provide health care services for urban Indians." Lack of accessible medical providers is an important issue in the Native American community. Most health care services provided by the Indian Health Service are provided in rural areas and on reservations. Indian Health Service provision is further complicated by the fact that more than 50 percent of Native Americans live in urban areas. Financing health care for the Native American community is a significant problem, despite the federal government's treaty agreements to provide health care for American Indians and Alaska Natives from federally recognized tribes. The impact of appropriation authorization over time on health disparities among clients of the Indian Health Service is an issue that needs to be explored formally by health disparity researchers. The Indian Health Service appropriations are divided into two budget categories—health services and health facilities. The federal government considers the provision of these services a trust responsibility based on federal statutes, treaties, court decisions, executive actions, and the Constitution, which assigns authority over Indian relations to Congress. Congress, however, has only a moral obligation, not a legal one, to Indian health care. The Supreme Court has rejected the idea that Indian Health Service is under any obligation to provide specific health program to Indians (U.S. Statutes at Large). In chapter 2, there is an extensive discussion of the impact of the Indian Health Service appropriations on Oklahoma's struggle to fund Medicaid.

The population served by the Indian Health Service has the highest rates of morbidity and mortality of all populations in the United States, that is, the greatest burden of health disparities. The availability of longitudinal data on appropriations and health indices create the opportunity for specific analyses to estimate the effect of appropriations on health disparities. How much of a decrease in death and illness could we observe if Indian Health Service facilities, services, and personnel were funded at originally proposed levels? What if a comparison is made between the Veterans Health Administration and the Indian Health Service? What could we learn about the association between resources and health outcomes? Many of the Indian Health Service facilities are located in rural communities. These same communities contain critical access hospitals, which are funded through Medicare. The co-localization of these facilities represents a modern-day example of racial segregation. The issue of separate but equal was ruled unsustainable by the Supreme Court during *Brown v. Topeka Board of Education*. Perhaps it is time to revisit this issue with the Indian Health Service and health care inequity.

## Public Law 106-525: Minority Health and Health Research and Education Act of 2000

The law has five titles that specify the creation of a National Institutes of Health–based center (Title I); guidelines for Health Disparities by the Agency for Healthcare Research and Quality (Title II); a study and report to Congress by the National Science Foundation (Title III); a component focused on Health Professions Education (Title IV); and a directive to engage in Public Awareness and Information Dissemination Campaign (Title V). There is also specific statutory language defining minority individuals. The National Center on Minority Health and Health Disparities (NCMHD) was established by the passage of the Minority Health and Health Disparities Research and Education Act of 2000. Public Law 106-525 was signed by President Clinton on November 22, 2000. Dr. John Ruffin was sworn in as the first director of the NCMHD in 2001. Programs mandated by Congress were implemented to expand the infrastructure of both intramural (NIH) and extramural institutions (colleges and universities) committed to health disparity research and to encourage the recruitment and retention of highly qualified minority and other scientists in the fields of biomedical, clinical, behavioral, and health services research. In 2002, the first National Advisory Council of the NCMHD was convened.

The origins of NCMHD can be traced back to 1990 when the Office of Research on Minority Health (ORMH) was established by the NIH director. Two years later, the Minority Health Initiative (MHI), a centerpiece of the ORMH agenda, was launched and initially funded at 45 million dollars. In 1993 Congress enacted Public Law 103-43, the Health Revitalization Act of 1993, to establish the Office of Research on Minority Health in the Office of the Director, National Institutes of Health. In 1997, the Advisory Committee on Research on Minority Health was established providing advice to the ORMH director and the NIH director, on research and research training with respect to minority health issues.

By 2003, the ORMH issued the first NIH Strategic Research Plan and Budget to Reduce and Ultimately Eliminate Health Disparities. What impact has this governmental initiative had on statistical measure of health disparity? In other words, how large were the gaps in death and illness prior to this law's enactment? Has there been a downward trend in key indicators of health over the past eight years? The Center's highest priority is support across all National Institutes of Health units with an emphasis on interinstitute funding of research. The National Institutes of Health is organized around categories of diseases or organ systems—the National Eye Institute, the National Cancer Institute, and the National Institute for Heart, Lung, and Blood. Is there evidence that this disease-specific approach to eliminating health disparities is yielding results? All government agencies are dependent on final appropriations to have the resources necessary to complete their stated mission. What is happening with appropriations for NCMHD? In the financial year 2008, appropriations were

9 percent less than requested. This downward trend in appropriations and the overall productivity of this center is worth watching because it reflects the commitment of the U.S. government to improve the health of its minority populations. As this center matures, will it survive several presidential transitions? Now that ACA has promoted the center to full institute status, will it continue its mission? The Cultural and Linguistically Appropriate Standards (CLAS) are one example of pioneering work from this center. What will the coming years bring?

## PROSPECTIVE STUDIES AND NEWLY ENACTED LEGISLATION

A confluence of factors has created the *political will* to create new laws with the potential to diminish health disparities. Prospective studies are designed to capture historic change as it is evolving. This section is designed to alert researchers to the potential for prospective studies of two new laws as they are implemented.

### Public Law 110–343, §511, and §512: Paul Wellstone and Pete Dominici Act

### Mental Health Parity and Addiction Equity Act of 2008 (Toxic Assets Relief Plan or TARP)

In the fall of 2008, U.S. banks with subprime interest mortgages required stabilization with federal dollars. This legislation came to be known as the Toxic Assets Relief Plan. A law to create equity in insurance markets between financial management of physical and mental illness was embedded within the TARP legislation. To honor the work of Senator Paul Wellstone and Senator Pete Dominici, Congress passed an amendment bearing their names to create parity in treatment, payment, and other features of mental illness and placing these services on par with the treatment of physical illnesses. Title V (subtitle B) §512 amends section 712 of the Employment Retirement Income Security Act of 1974. It requires group health insurance plans to provide benefits for mental illness and substance abuse treatment that are comparable to covered treatments for physical illnesses. The legislative language goes into considerable detail describing the timeline for phasing in these provisions and employer requirements for financing. Provisions of this law became active beginning in 2010. Do these provisions influence mental illness treatment access for men and women in the workplace and for racial and ethnic groups who are employed in similar positions? In short, what does this legislation do to diminish mental health disparity? Are there unintended consequences for loss of employment among persons who utilize these benefits? Are these consequences differentially experienced by racial and ethnic groups? Is there evidence of resistance to its implementation by employers?

## Public Law 111–03: The American Revitalization and Reinvestment Act (ARRA, The Stimulus Package)

To accurately assess the true extent of health disparities across racial and ethnic groups we must, examine data collected by the Centers for Medicare and Medicaid. The ARRA contained the following section: *§3002(b)(2)(vii) The use of electronic systems to ensure the comprehensive collection of patient demographic data, including, at a minimum, race, ethnicity, primary language, and gender information.* This new data element will create the opportunity to measure disparities in death and illness at multiple levels—by geographic areas, zip code, and health care institution. For the first time, researchers will be able to compare hospitals and clinics within a city to measure accessibility by disadvantaged groups and to detect differences in treatment outcome.

## SUMMARY

Science contributes to our understanding of health care inequity and disparity. Analyses of newly enacted legislation cannot be left to historians. In the United States, each new health care law has measurable effects. ACA creates the tools necessary to measure changes *as they happen*. The Vital Health Statistics System is a surveillance network that operates primarily through our public health infrastructure. The public health infrastructure has the Centers for Disease Control and Prevention (CDC) at the top. It monitors the minority health through mortality reports and surveys. Regional variation in the quality of health care delivery is a poorly understood part of the path leading to disparity. ACA extends the ability of the CDC to monitor this pathway. With the use of these new data, researchers will have the tools needed to study the effect of new legislation on existing health disparity.

## BIBLIOGRAPHY

Aapro, M., M. Extermann, and L. Repetto. "Evaluation of the Elderly with Cancer." *Annals of Oncology* 11 (2000): 223–29.

American Cancer Society. "American Cancer Society Guidelines for the Early Detection of Cancer," http://www.cancer.org/Healthy/FindCancerEarly/ CancerScreeningGuidelines/american-cancer-society-guidelines-for-the-early-detection-of-cancer.

American College of Physicians. "Screening for Prostate Cancer." *Annals of Internal Medicine* 126, no. 6 (1997): 480–4.

American Urological Association. "Prostate-Specific Antigen (PSA) Best Practice Policy." *Oncology* 14, no. 2 (2000): 267.

Bach, Peter B., Hoangmai H. Pham, Deborah Schrag, Ramsey C. Tate, and J. Lee Hargraves. "Primary Care Physicians Who Treat Blacks and Whites." *New England Journal of Medicine* 351, no. 6 (2004): 575–84.

Blackwell, Debra L., Mark D. Hayward, and Eileen M. Crimmins. "Does Childhood Health Affect Chronic Morbidity in Later Life?" *Social Science & Medicine* 52 (2001): 1269–84.

Borer, J. G., J. Sherman, M. C. Solomon, M. W. Plawker, and R. J. Macchia. "Age Specific Prostate Specific Antigen Reference Ranges: Population Specific." *Journal of Urology* 159, no. 2 (1998): 444–48.

Bureau of Economic Analysis, U.S. Department of Commerce. Survey of Current Business Online, 2009. Published electronically February 2009, http://www.bea.gov/scb/pdf/2009/02%20February/0209_healthcare.pdf.

Byrd, W. Michael, and Linda A. Clayton. *An American Health Dilemma: Race, Medicine, and Health Care in the United States 1900–2000.* New York: Routledge, 2002.

Byrne, Julianne, Larry G. Kessler, and Susan S. Devesa. "The Prevalence of Cancer among Adults in the United States: 1987." *Cancer* 69, no. 8 (1992): 2154–59.

Capocaccia, R., and R. De Angelis. "Estimating the Completeness of Prevalence Based on Cancer Registry Data." *Statistics in Medicine* 16, no. 4 (1997): 425–40.

Catalona, William J., Deborah S. Smith, Timothy L. Ratliff, Kathy M. Dodds, Douglas E. Coplen, Jerry J. J. Yuan, John A. Petros, and Gerald L. Andriole. "Measurement of Prostate-Specific Antigen in Serum as a Screening Test for Prostate Cancer." *New England Journal of Medicine* 324, no. 17 (1991): 1156–61.

Catalona, W. J., D. S. Smith, T. L. Ratliff, and J. W. Basler. "Detection of Organ-Confined Prostate Cancer Is Increased through Prostate-Specific Antigen-Based Screening." *Journal of American Medical Association* 270, no. 8 (1993): 948–54.

Catalona, W. J., J. P. Richie, F. R. Ahmann, M. A. Hudson, P. T. Scardino, R. C. Flanigan, J. B. deKernion, T. L. Ratliff, L. R. Kavoussi, B. L. Dalkin, et al. "Comparison of Digital Rectal Examination and Serum Prostate Specific Antigen in the Early Detection of Prostate Cancer: Results of a Multicenter Clinical Trial of 6,630 Men." *Journal of Urology* 151, no. 5 (1994): 1283–90.

Centers for Disease Control and Prevention (CDC). "Cancer Registries: The Foundation for Cancer Prevention and Control. Fact Sheet from the Division of Cancer Prevention and Control." Department of Health and Human Services, 2011.

Centers for Disease Control and Prevention (CDC). "Screening with the Prostate-Specific Antigen Test—Texas, 1997." *Morbidity and Mortality Weekly Report (MMWR)* 49, no. 36 (2000): 818–20.

Centers for Disease Control and Prevention (CDC). "Recent Trends in Mortality Rates for Four Major Cancers, by Sex and Race/Ethnicity—United States, 1990–1998." *Morbidity and Mortality Weekly Report* 51 (2002): 49–53.

Chodak, G.W., P. Keller, and H.W. Schoenberg. "Assessment of Screening for Prostate Cancer Using the Digital Rectal Examination." *Journal of Urology* 141, no. 5 (1989): 1136–38.

Chute, C.G., L.A. Panser, C.J. Girman, J.E. Oesterling, H.A. Guess, S.J. Jacobsen, and M.M. Lieber. "The Prevalence of Prostatism: A Population-Based Survey of Urinary Symptoms." *Journal of Urology* 150, no. 1 (1993): 85–89.

Cooner, W.H., B.R. Mosley, C.L. Rutherford Jr., J.H. Beard, H.S. Pond, W.J. Terry, T.C. Iqel, and D.D. Kidd. "Prostate Cancer Detection in a Clinical Urological Practice by Ultrasonography, Digital Rectal Examination and Prostate Specific Antigen." *Journal of Urology* 143 (1990): 1146–52 (discussion: 52–54).

Coughlin, Teresa, Timothy Waidmann, and Molly O'Malley Watts. "Where Does the Burden Lie? Medicaid and Medicare Spending for Dual Eligible Beneficiaries." Kaiser Commission on Medicaid and the Uninsured, Kaiser Family Foundation, Washington, DC, 2009.

Crawford, E.D., D. Chia, G.L. Andriole, Douglas Redding, Edward P. Gelmann, John K. Gohagan, Paul Pinsky, Richard B. Hayes, David L. Levin, Richard M. Fagerstrom, and Barnett S. Kramer. "PSA Testing Interval Reduction in Screening Intervals: Data from the Prostate, Lung, Colorectal and Ovarian Cancer (PLCO) Screening Trial." Paper presented at the ASCO Annual Meeting, 2002.

Crimmins, Eileen M., Mark D. Hayward, and Yasuhiko Saito. "Changing Mortality and Morbidity Rates and the Health Status and Life Expectancy of the Older Population." *Demography* 31, no. 1 (1994): 159–75.

Crimmins, Eileen M., Mark D. Hayward, and Yasuhiko Saito. "Differentials in Active Life Expectancy in the Older Population of the United States." *The Journals of Gerontology Series B: Psychological Sciences and Social Sciences* 51B, no. 3 (1996): S111–S20.

Crimmins, Eileen M., Mark D. Hayward, Yasuhiko Saito, M. Johnston, M. Hayward, and T. Seeman. "Age Differences in Allostatic Load: An Index of Physiological Dysregulation." *Experimental Gerontology* 38, no. 7 (2003): 731–34.

De Angelis G., R. De Angelis, L. Frova, and A. Verdecchia. "MIAMOD: A Computer Package to Estimate Chronic Disease Morbidity Using Mortality and Survival Data." *Computer Methods and Programs in Biomedicine* 44, no. 2 (1994): 99–107.

Dunn, Andrew S., Kanan V. Shridharani, Wendy Lou, Jeffrey Bernstein, and Carol R. Horowitz. "Physician–Patient Discussions of Controversial Cancer Screening Tests." *American Journal of Preventive Medicine* 20, no. 2 (2001): 130–34.

"Early Prostate Cancer: What You Should Know." *American Family Physician* 71, no. 10 (2005): 1929–30.

Feldman, A.R., L. Kessler, M.H. Myers, M.D. Naughton. "The Prevalence of Cancer. Estimates Based on the Connecticut Tumor Registry." *New England Journal of Medicine* 315, no. 22 (1986): 1394–97.

Fox, Maggie. "United States Hospital Profits Fall to Zero: Thomson Reuters." *Reuters,* 2009. Published electronically March 2, 2009, http://www.reuters.com/article/2009/03/02/us-hospitals-usa-idUSTRE5216G320090302.

Gail, M.H., L. Kessler, D. Midthune, and S. Scoppa. "Two Approaches for Estimating Disease Prevalence from Population-Based Registries of Incidence and Total Mortality." *Biometrics* 55, no. 4 (1999): 1137–44.

Giles, G. "How Important Are Estimates of Cancer Prevalence?" *Annals of Oncology* 13, no. 6 (2002): 815–16.

Government Accounting Office Legislative History. PL 79-725.

Hayward, Mark D., Eileen M. Crimmins, Toni P. Miles, and Yu Yang. "The Significance of Socioeconomic Status in Explaining the Gap in Chronic Health Conditions." *American Sociological Review* 65 (2000): 910–30.

Hayward, Mark D., Eileen M. Crimmins, Toni P. Miles, Yu Yang, T.P. Miles, F.P. Stafford, et al. "Living Longer, Staying Well: Promoting Good Health for Older Americans." Paper presented at the Congressional Briefing, Washington, DC, 2001.

Jacobsen, S.J., E.J. Bergstralh, H.A. Guess, S.K. Katusic, G.G. Klee, J.E. Oesterling, and M.M. Lieber. "Predictive Properties of Serum-Prostate-Specific Antigen Testing in a Community-Based Setting." *Archives of Internal Medicine* 156, no. 21 (1996): 2462–68.

Kaiser Family Foundation. "Medicare Spending and Financing Fact Sheet." Kaiser Family Foundation Program on Medicare Policy, 2009, http://www.kff.org/medicare/upload/7305-06.pdf.

Kappler, Charles J. *Indian Affairs: Laws & Treaties,* edited by Charles J. Kappler. Vol. 1–7. Washington Government Printing Office, 1904–1979.

Kim, K. "Improving the Health of Older Asian Women." Paper presented at the Improving the Health of Older Women of Color Conference, Palo Alto, December 10–11, 2004.

Majette, G. R. "Access to Health Care: What a Difference Shade of Color Make." *Annals of Health Law* 12, no. 1 (2003): 121–42.

Mariotto, A., A. Gigli, R. Capocaccia, A. Tavilla, L. X. Clegg, M. Depry, S. Scoppa, L.A.G. Ries, J. H. Rowland, G. Tesauro, and E. J. Feuer. "Complete and Limited Duration Cancer Prevalence Estimates," http://seer.cancer.gov/csr/1973_1999/.

Marwick, C. "ACS Sets Blueprint for Action against Prostate Cancer in African Americans." *Journal of the American Medical Association* 279, no. 6 (1998): 418–19.

Merrill, Ray M., Riccardo Capocaccia, Eric J. Feuer, and Angela Mariotto. "Cancer Prevalence Estimates Based on Tumour Registry Data in the Surveillance, Epidemiology, and End Results (Seer) Program." *International Journal of Epidemiology* 29, no. 2 (2000): 197–207.

Micheli, A., E. Mugno, V. Krogh, et al. "Europreval Working Group: Cancer Prevalence in European Registry Areas." *Annals of Oncology* 13 (2002): 840–65.

Miles, Toni P., and David McBride. "World War I Origins of the Syphilis Epidemic among 20th Century Black Americans: A Biohistorical Analysis." *Social Science Medicine* 45, no. 1 (1997): 61–69.

Miles, Toni P., and J. Bland. "Rates of Multiple Primary Malignant Neoplasms in Older Adults: Seer 1989–1999." Paper presented at the 7th International Society of Geriatric Oncology Cancer in the Elderly, Boston, MA, September 27–28, 2002.

Monson, K., D.A. Litvak, and R. J. Bold. "Surgery and the Older Patient: Surgical Oncology." *Archives of Surgery* 138 (2003): 1061–67.

Murray, Christopher J.L., Sandeep C. Kulkarni, Catherine Michaud, Niels Tomihima, Maria T. Bulzacchelli, Terrell J. Landiorio, and Majid Ezzati. "Eight Americas: Investigating Mortality Disparities across Races, Counties, and Race-Counties in the United States." *PLoS Medicine* 3, no. 9 (2006): e260. Published electronically September 12, 2006, http://www.plosmedicine.org/article/info:doi/10.1371/journal.pmed.0030260.

Naitoh, John, Rebecca L. Zeiner, and Jean B. Dekernion. "Diagnosis and Treatment of Prostate Cancer." *American Family Physician* 57, no. 7 (1998): 1531–39.

National Cancer Institute. "Cancer Health Disparities: Fact Sheet." Updated April 4, 2003, http://www.cancer.gov/cancertopics/disparities.

Nusbaum, N. J. "Rehabilitation and the Older Cancer Patient." *American Journal of the Medical Sciences* 327 (2004): 86–90.

Office of the Federal Register. *United States Statutes at Large*. Boston: Little, Brown and Company, 1851–69.

Office of the Federal Register. *United States Statutes at Large*. Washington, DC: U.S. Government Printing Office, 1875–present.

Optenberg, S. A., and I. M. Thompson. "Economics of Screening for Carcinoma of the Prostate." *Urologic Clinics of North America* 17, no. 4 (1990): 719–37.

Pear, Robert. "Many Doctors Shun Patients with Medicare." *New York Times,* 2002. Published electronically March 17, 2002, http://www.nytimes.com/2002/03/17/us/many-doctors-shun-patients-with-medicare.html?pagewanted=all&src=pm.

Rosenberg, J., and E. Small. "Prostate Cancer Update." *Current Opinion in Oncology* 15 (2003): 217–21.

Rowland, D., and B. Lyons. "Medicare, Medicaid, and the Elderly Poor." *Health Care Financing* Winter 18, no. 2 (1996): 61–85.

Scott, Morey S. "AUA Issues a Policy Report on PSA Monitoring. The American Urological Association." *American Family Physician* 62, no. 4 (2000): 883–84.

Shavers, Vickie L., and Martin L. Brown. "Racial and Ethnic Disparities in the Receipt of Cancer Treatment." *Journal of the National Cancer Institute* 94, no. 5 (2002): 334–57.

Skinner, J., and W. Zhou. "Public Policy and Income Distribution." *The Measurement and Evolution of Health Inequality: Evidence from the United States Medicare Population.*, edited by A. J. Auerbach, D. Card, and J. M. Quigley. Chapter 7. New York: Russell Sage Foundation, 2006.

Thompson, Ian M., Donna K. Pauler, Phyllis J. Goodman, Catherine M. Tangen, M. Scott Lucia, Howard L. Parnes, Lori M. Minasian, et al. "Prevalence of Prostate Cancer among Men with a Prostate-Specific Antigen Level ≤ 4.0 ng Per Milliliter." *New England Journal of Medicine* 350, no. 22 (2004): 2239–46.

U.S. Cancer Statistics Working Group. "United States Cancer Statistics: 2001 Incidence and Mortality." Centers for Disease Control and Prevention and National Cancer Institute, Atlanta, GA, 2004.

U.S. Congress, 79th. "Interstate and Foreign Commerce Committee Report, House of Representatives, Report No. 2519," July 13, 1946.

U.S. Congress, 79th. "Education and Labor Committee Report, Senate Report No. 674, Volume 3: 1–21," October 30, 1945.

Verdecchia, Arduino, Riccardo Capocaccia, Viviana Egidi, and Antonio Golini. "A Method for the Estimation of Chronic Disease Morbidity and Trends from Mortality Data." *Statistics in Medicine* 8, no. 2 (1989): 201–16.

Vihko, P., M. Kontturi, O. Lukkarinen, J. Ervasti, and R. Vihko. "Screening for Carcinoma of the Prostate. Rectal Examination, and Enzymatic and Radioimmunologic Measurements of Serum Acid Phosphatase Compared." *Cancer* 56, no. 1 (1985): 173–77.

Volk, Robert J., and Alvah R. Cass. "The Accuracy of Primary Care Patients' Self-Reports of Prostate-Specific Antigen Testing." *American Journal of Preventive Medicine* 22, no. 1 (2002): 56–58.

Wailoo, Keith. *Dying in the City of the Blues: Sickle Cell Anemia and the Politics of Race and Health*. Chapel Hill: The University of North Carolina Press, 2001.

Walke, Roger. "Indian Health Service: Health Care Delivery, Status, Funding, and Legislative Issues (7-5700, Rl33022)." CRS Report for Congress, 57, Congressional Research Service, 2009.

Wolf, A.M., and D.M. Becker. "Cancer Screening and Informed Patient Discussions. Truth and Consequences." *Archives of Internal Medicine* 156, no. 10 (1996): 1069–72.

# Abbreviations

| | |
|---|---|
| ACA | (Patient Protection and) Affordable Care Act of 2010 |
| ACS | American Cancer Society |
| AEI | American Enterprise Institute |
| AMA | American Medical Association |
| BPCA | Best Pharmaceuticals for Children Act |
| BRT | Business Roundtable |
| CAH | critical access hospitals |
| CAHPS | Consumer Assessment of Healthcare Providers and Systems |
| CAIF | Coalition against Insurance Fraud |
| CAP | Center for American Progress |
| CDC | Centers for Disease Control and Prevention |
| CEO | chief executive officer |
| CHIP | Children's Health Insurance Program |
| CLAS | National Standards on Culturally and Linguistically Appropriate Services |
| CMS | Center for Medicare and Medicaid Services |
| COBRA | Consolidated Omnibus Budget Reconciliation Act |
| DAP | Dartmouth Atlas Project |
| DME | durable medical equipment |

| | |
|---|---|
| DSH | disproportionate share hospitals |
| FBI | Federal Bureau of Investigation |
| FCA | False Claims Act |
| FDA | Food and Drug Administration |
| FFS | fee-for-service |
| FHK | Foundation for a Healthy Kentucky |
| FPL | federal poverty level |
| FQHC | Federally Qualified Health Center |
| GAO | Government Accounting Office |
| Gen X | generation X |
| HBCUs | historically black colleges and universities |
| HCBS | home and community-based services |
| HEAT | Health Care Fraud Prevention and Enforcement Action Team |
| HEDIS | Health Care Effectiveness Data and Information Set |
| HHS | (U.S. Department of) Health and Human Services |
| Hill-Burton | Hill-Burton Hospital Survey and Construction Act of 1946 |
| HIPAA | Health Insurance Portability and Accountability Act |
| HLOGA | Honest Leadership and Open Government Act of 2007 |
| HSA | health savings account |
| IHS | Indian Health Service |
| MA Plans | Medicare Advantage Plans |
| MFP | Money Follows the Person |
| MFSF | Medicare Fraud Strike Force |
| MLR | medical loss ratio |
| MMIS | Medicaid Management Information System |
| MMNY | Medicaid Matters New York |
| NAACP | National Association for the Advancement of Colored People |
| NAAL | National Assessment of Adult Literacy |
| NAPH | National Association of Public Hospitals and Health Systems |

| NCD | national coverage determination |
| NCI | National Cancer Institute |
| NCLR | National Council of La Raza |
| NCQA | National Committee for Quality Assurance |
| NIH | National Institutes of Health |
| NQF | National Quality Forum |
| NSC | National Supplier Clearinghouse |
| OBRA | Omnibus Budget Reconciliation Act |
| OHCA | Oklahoma Health Care Authority |
| OMH | Office of Minority Health |
| PE | presumptive eligibility |
| PREA | Pediatric Research Equity Act |
| PSA | Prostate Specific Antigen |
| PTH | parathyroid hormone |
| SBP | single-benefit plans |
| SCI | Oklahoma Strategic Coverage Initiative |
| SRMC | Shasta Regional Medical Center |
| STD | sexually transmitted disease |
| TMD | The March of Dimes |
| VHA | Veterans Health Administration |
| VISN | Veterans Integrated Service Networks |
| WHO | World Health Organization |

# Index

# About the Author

**Toni P. Miles,** MD, PhD, is the director of the Institute of Gerontology and a professor of epidemiology and biostatistics in the College of Public Health, both at the University of Georgia-Athens. Dr. Miles was inspired to write this book during her American Political Science Association Congressional Fellowship in 2009 while serving as a staff member on the U.S. Senate Finance Committee during the development of the Affordable Care Act. She continues to assist state agencies and professional organizations as they implement various components of the landmark health reform legislation of 2010. She has authored more than 120 scientific publications in gerontology, epidemiology, and minority health and has served as editor for a number of volumes on gerontology. She lives in Athens, Georgia, with her husband of 39 years.